Breastfeeding Does Suck: Tips, Tricks & Knowledge for a Great Experience

By Mindy Cockeram

Copyright ©2019 Mindy Cockeram

ISBN-9781790662302

Cover design by Julie Cary

Legal Disclaimer

The information provided in this book is designed to provide helpful information on the subjects discussed. This book is not meant to be used, nor should it be used, to diagnose or treat any medical condition. For diagnosis or treatment of any medical problem, consult your own physician. The author is not responsible for any specific health needs that may require medical supervision and is not liable for any damages or negative consequences from any treatment, action, application or preparation, to any person reading or following the information in this book. References are provided for informational purposes only and do not constitute endorsement of any websites or other sources. Readers should be aware that the websites listed in this book may change.

Acknowledgments

This book is possible solely because of the wonderful women, partners, teachers, doulas, midwives, pediatricians and lactation consultants I have met in my journey through breastfeeding education – both in the UK and the USA. Educators in the UK's National Childbirth Trust & National Health Service, Kaiser Permanente, Lamaze International and the Inland Empire Breastfeeding Coalition have been instrumental in their support and help. A special thanks to Jessica, Sharlene, Kayellen, Holly, Mia and Tamika. Thanks also to my family and friends who encourage me to continue writing. I also couldn't have done it without Corinne, Emmeline and all the moms who shared their breastfeeding experiences with me. Thank you!

Mindy Cockeram

Contents

*Chapter specifically designated for partners to read

INTRODUCTION

UNLOCKING TIPS, TRICKS & KNOWLEDGE!

Breastfeeding is a daunting prospect. The rebel in me wanted to skip breastfeeding altogether just because I felt so pressured. At birth, 81.1% (CDC, 2016) of women start out breastfeeding, 15% quit before hospital discharge and only 32.4% of women reach their breastfeeding goals. I don't think that anyone can argue that breast milk isn't the best milk for your baby but we all know a woman who struggled with painful bleeding nipples or milk supply issues and gave up. Just like labor, success in breastfeeding is a psychological, emotional and physical journey. Preparing for that journey ahead of time is a great first step in conquering fear.

There are lots of tips, tricks and learning points that can make breastfeeding successful – or at least reduce the chance of failure. If my mother knew back then what I know now about breastfeeding, I'm convinced she would have been successful. By talking to hundreds of breastfeeding mothers, reading evidence based research, studying the anatomy and physiology of the breast and dissecting feeding issues, I realize that there are many things a woman and her care provider can do to make breastfeeding easier. This book is about sharing all that knowledge with you.

There are also several choices a woman can opt for that make breastfeeding harder (!) although I've never met anyone who intentionally did so on purpose – all decisions were taken with the best of intentions for all concerned. It is sometimes only in hindsight that we realize that some problems could have been avoided or more choices could have been explored in order to improve an outcome. Hopefully this book will help you see those options through the windshield instead of the rear view mirror.

In breastfeeding, as in life, knowledge is power. Knowledge allows choices. And knowledge reduces fear. Also, partners who receive breastfeeding education tend to support the new mother better and improve her chances of success, so encourage yours to read the chapters I've flagged with the designation *(PARTNER*)*. If you want to review a chapter quickly, I've included a summary at the end of each one. Many chapters also have a Breastfeeding Story that explores or highlights the main points of that chapter.

Before we talk about ways to make breastfeeding successful, let's look at my reverse psychology list. Here are several ways I know of to make breastfeeding quite the opposite.

HOW TO MAKE BREASTFEEDING FAIL:

☐ Be fearful of breastfeeding and remain tense when feeding the baby. Don't make a breastfeeding plan.

☐ Know nothing about how labor and postpartum decisions or drugs can affect breastfeeding or delay milk flow.

☐ Know nothing about how the breast works to produce milk.

☐ Expect the baby to gain weight quickly in the first few days and quit breastfeeding if he/she doesn't.

☐ If you need to give a supplement of formula, don't return to breastfeeding.

☐ Wait until a baby is crying to feed him or her.

☐ Use uncomfortable positions during feeds.

☐ Eat, drink or use whatever food and drugs you want without knowing their effect on lactation.

☐ Don't use any pumps or lactation aids.

☐ Ignore problems until they become emergencies.

☐ Have no one you can turn to for help, support and a spare set of hands.

☐ Stop breastfeeding without considering other options.

The rest of this book is dedicated to unravelling everything I have learned as an educator in order to make your experience of breastfeeding as successful as possible. I will also walk you through the various benefits and risks of many decisions you may have to make about specific breastfeeding topics.

PREACHING TO THE CONVERTED

Most breastfeeding books will spend at least a chapter acquainting you with the benefits of breastfeeding and I have summarized some of those wonderful benefits on the next page. I've kept it short because I figure that if you have gone through the trouble of reading this far, you are already thinking that *breast feeding is best feeding* if you can manage it. I think it's also fair to understand the risks (or downsides) so that you are able to plan for success. Breastfeeding is more of a **lifestyle** than it is a process and getting mentally prepared for what you need to do is a useful exercise. Here's a quick overview of the benefits and risks.

BENEFITS OF BREASTFEEDING:

- ❖ There is a deep joy and great level of satisfaction for the mother once she has mastered breastfeeding
- ❖ Healthier mother (lowers chances of breast and ovarian cancer and diabetes) and baby (less likely to develop diabetes, asthma, Inflammatory Bowel Diseases, allergies, ADHD, SIDS, childhood obesity and enhances brain development)
- ❖ Boosts babies immune system
- ❖ Saves approximately $2000+ per year
- ❖ Helps mother burn calories and shrink uterus back to pre-pregnancy size
- ❖ Increases the maternal nurturing bond
- ❖ Safer than using artificial baby milk
- ❖ Increases mother's self esteem
- ❖ *and HUNDREDS of other benefits*

RISKS OF BREASTFEEDING:

- ➢ You must either be with your baby at all feeding times or able to pump what your baby would normally remove from your breast at every feed 24 hours a day
- ➢ Breastfeeding can limit some job opportunities and life or work experiences
- ➢ Feeding from the breast or pumping is time consuming and requires dedication

➤ Some women struggle with latch issues, soreness and nipple or areola damage

➤ Failure to breastfeed can cause emotional distress and feelings of guilt or failure for the mother

You can see that the benefits seemingly outweigh the risks by a wide margin. Getting a baby off to the best physiological start in life by breastfeeding may be of utmost importance to some mothers while others may rank personal achievement, personal health or financial wealth as more important *overall*. The most important goal is to ***feed the baby and keep him or her alive and thriving – regardless of breast or bottle***. But as I said, I think I'm talking to an audience who has already decided to give breastfeeding a try.

Read on and let me know how your breastfeeding experience goes. I am always looking for a good feeding story to reduce fear and motivate others at *Learn4Birth*'s *Facebook page* or at www.learn4birth.com. Good luck and good skill for successful breastfeeding. Enjoy the journey.

CHAPTER 1

LOSE THE FEAR OF NOT BEING ABLE TO BREASTFEED

BREASTFEEDING DOESN'T HAVE TO SUCK if you lose the fear of not being able to do so. Women are not born with breastfeeding skills; they learn them. Creating a breastfeeding plan, having good support from the start and becoming educated about breastfeeding will empower you.

WERE YOU BORN IN CAPTIVITY?

My Lactation Instructor told our class an incredible story about a female gorilla born in an Ohio Zoo that didn't know how to breastfeed. I always thought that breastfeeding was instinctive; how could this be true? The gorilla had been born in captivity and had never seen any other gorillas feeding their babies. She had no innate instinct to put her baby to the breast. When her first baby was born, she had no idea what to do. The crying baby left the gorilla feeling helpless and stressed. The baby gorilla died.

When the zookeeper found out the same gorilla was pregnant again a year later, he called on the members of the local La Leche League (LLL) for help. The La Leche League is a volunteer organization that promotes and supports breastfeeding. Several mothers brought their infants to the zoo and sat breastfeeding in front of the gorilla enclosure. By watching the breastfeeding mothers, the gorilla realized that latching the baby on to her breast was the way to stop the infant from crying and keep it alive!

While babies are born with an innate searching and sucking instinct, mothers are not born with breastfeeding skills. If, like the great Ohio gorilla, you never saw your mother, aunts, sisters or friends breastfeeding, it is most likely a skill that you too will have to learn. At least you know where to start.

CHOOSE THREE WORDS

I always ask women to write down three words that describe the kind of breastfeeding experience they'd like to have on yellow stickies. Then I stick them up on the wall to justify every activity we do (and every chapter in this book). So have a think. What three words describe the way you'd like to feel when breastfeeding or how you'd like breastfeeding to be?

1.

2.

3.

I've never had anyone say they wanted sore nipples, a painful latch or a low supply. The most common words written to describe the kind of experience women want are easy, pain-free and successful – a bit like birth. Here are some of the common responses:

WHAT KIND OF BREASTFEEDING DO YOU WANT?
* Easy * Pain-free * Natural * Healthy * Dignified * Civilized * Textbook * Happy * In-control * Not scared * Remarkable * Normal * Well Supported* Lotsa Milk * Successful * Calorie burning * Best for Baby * 1 Year *

Now that you've chosen some words to use as goals, you need to plan a strategy. I view breastfeeding plans a bit like a satellite navigation system. First you need to pick your destination; then you need to work out the directions (i.e. how you aim to achieve it). You can never be sure which route the *system* is going to take you and occasionally a road gets closed with no notice but it's pretty certain you'll arrive at the other end one way or another.

Writing a breastfeeding plan can be a little tricky because it needs to be written with the hospital's and employer's policies in mind from the start. For example, you can't plan on having the baby skin to skin immediately if you have a C-Section and your hospital restrains your arms during the operation. You also need to consider when and how breastfeeding and pumping will work when you go back to school or employment. Will you have a chance to pump at work? Do they have a refrigerator you can store breastmilk in? Can you get home in time for the 6-7pm feed?

You may find that the strategy of a breastfeeding plan is not something you can write clearly now. I put it in the first chapter to plant a seed but it is probably best to wait until the middle of the 3rd trimester to begin formulating exactly what strategies you will use – based on your own medical situation, your relationship with your care provider, when you are returning to work or school and what you have learned about making breastfeeding easier.

USE FLEXIBLE LANGUAGE

As I say to my kids all the time, there is a big difference between the words 'would like' and 'want' – especially on a breastfeeding plan. Inflexible language can be interpreted as passionate but could also be interpreted as *stubborn, unrealistic or difficult* in a clinical setting. What follows is an excerpt from a breastfeeding plan written by a passionate woman who wanted to breastfeed for a year. Imagine how she'd feel rereading it if she ended up having a C-Section, wasn't able to hold the baby for three hours and then quit breastfeeding after two days?

Our Three Goals for Breastfeeding:

1. **Breastfeed exclusively for one year**

2. **Do not use formula for any reason**

3. **Learn to pump immediately**

Breastfeeding Plan:

- ➢ Do not allow anything but breastmilk for baby
- ➢ No C-Section (which could hinder breastfeeding)
- ➢ In labor, allow no IV fluids for hydration
- ➢ In labor, have an epidural instead of a narcotic if needed
- ➢ Make sure my partner supports my breastfeeding decisions
- ➢ Do not let staff force formula on my baby
- ➢ Remember that I am capable of breastfeeding a child

The wording of this breastfeeding plan may cause stress between the mother and anybody who reads it for many reasons. First, this plan makes an assumption that she will have a normal, vaginal birth. Her plan to have an epidural instead of a narcotic contradicts not receiving an IV for fluids since most hospitals won't offer an epidural unless the mother has received 1000cc of fluid through an IV. It also assumes that she will be able to pump and will have no need to supplement (give a little extra) with formula. Finally, it suggests a distrust of her care providers.

In Labor and Delivery, doctors and nurses are paid to manage the labor and can be very forthright in making sure policies are enforced and their clinical advice is followed. Having said that, you will find that most hospital staff is very keen to help new mothers breastfeed and avoid formula unless there is a true medical reason. Here is a revised excerpt with flexible language and realistic expectations:

<u>Our Three Goals for Breastfeeding:</u>

1. Breastfeed exclusively for ~~one year~~ as long as it works for mother and baby

2. ~~Do not use formula for any reason~~ Consider supplementing for true medical reason(s)

3. Learn to ~~pump efficiently~~ remove milk from the breast in as many ways as possible

---

Breastfeeding Plan:

➤ ~~Do not allow anything but breastmilk for baby~~ Aim to breastfeed as long as possible and get help if struggling

➤ ~~No C-Section (which could hinder breastfeeding)~~ Work towards a normal vaginal birth by following *Cut Your Labor in Half: 19 Secrets to a Faster and Easier Birth (available on amazon.com)*

➤ ~~In labor, allow no IV fluids for hydration~~ In labor, hydrate by mouth if/until no longer possible

➤ ~~In labor, have an epidural instead of a narcotic if needed~~ Avoid any medications that could affect the baby's latch or my milk supply

➤ ~~Make sure~~ Have partner attend breastfeeding class or read Partner Chapters so that he/she is educated and supports my decisions ~~my partner supports my breastfeeding decisions~~

➤ ~~Do not~~ Let staff ~~force formula on my baby~~ help by explaining the benefits and risks of any decisions that need to be made and demonstrate hand expressing with me

➤ Remember that I am capable of breastfeeding a child

From the tone of the revised plan, a care provider can tell that the mother is prepared, knowledgeable, flexible and understands the challenges she may face. Remember, breastfeeding plans cannot usually be executed in isolation from your care providers. The hospital staff wants you and your baby to be healthy and thrive.

CHOOSE A 'BABY FRIENDLY' HOSPITAL

Where you choose to give birth is an important first step in initiating successful breastfeeding. If you are well supported in the first few hours and days after the birth, you will be much more likely to keep going and seek help if you need it. Across the United States, roughly 25% of hospitals have the designation 'Baby Friendly' (BFHI). This means they have gone through a rigorous staff training program and will encourage breastfeeding over artificial baby milk. According to **www.babyfriendlyusa.org**, hospitals with this designation believe:

> (1) human milk fed through direct breastfeeding is the
> optimal way for human infants to be nurtured and nourished;
> (2) the precious first days should be protected as a time of
> bonding and support not influenced by commercial interests;
> and (3) every mother should be informed about the benefits
> of breastfeeding and respected to make her own choice.

You may not have a hospital in your area (yet) with the Baby Friendly designation but if there is one within a reasonable distance, choosing to birth further afield may improve breastfeeding success. You can find BFHI Hospitals using the locator at **www.babyfriendlyusa.org**.

PRESUME YOU WILL BE ABLE TO BREASTFEED

Women encounter problems that can render milk-making or breastfeeding difficult or occasionally impossible. Speak to a lactation consultant before the baby is born if you have doubts or questions about your physical ability to breastfeed. For the time being, let's presume you will be able to breastfeed! Don't make assumptions about your own abilities just because your mother, sister, friend or neighbor could not breastfeed. Stay positive about your abilities.

In Chapter 3, we will explore how many medications, decisions and interventions in labor may hinder early breastfeeding. In Chapter 10, we will cover conditions or situations which may render women unable to breastfeed with ease or occasionally not at all. Finally in Chapter 12, we will explain pumps, devices and equipment which can assist the breastfeeding mother in many ways.

KEEP READING (AND LEARNING)

Learning about breastfeeding seems finite. Surely after reading a few chapters, you should know all you need to know. While that may be the case, I can't tell you how much I have learned from listening to other mothers long after I thought I knew more than anyone in the room about breastfeeding. Besides this book, find out (in advance) what breastfeeding support groups are near you, who to call in the middle of the night if you have an issue and which of your friends and family members breastfed their kids. The latter can support you if you get discouraged or troubled. Women who have bottle fed formula to their kids are probably going to struggle to support you.

New equipment and technology appear all the time and can change the goalposts of breastfeeding. In the last few years, apps like *Wonder Weeks* and products like the *Haakaa* have helped countless mothers link baby behavior to new developmental milestones and collect milk drops with ease. Recently I learned about a rare bacterium (Serratia marcescens) that turns the mother's breastmilk pink and causes severe illness for both the mother and child from a TV show about unusual cases in the Emergency Room. Keep your eyes open daily for new research and news on breastfeeding. You can never have enough information and medicine evolves constantly.

SUMMARY:

☐ Breastfeeding is a learned skill and becomes a lifestyle choice.

☐ Babies are born with an instinct to suck but mothers are not born with breastfeeding knowledge. It will take time to learn how to breastfeed effectively.

☐ Pinpointing three words that would describe your ideal breastfeeding experience is a good starting point.

☐ Breastfeeding plans are a useful tool for thinking through your goals and strategies. If you write one, keep it flexible and make certain that your birth partner(s) knows how to support the plan.

☐ Choose a Baby Friendly (BFHI) Hospital if there is one within reach. Also, understand your hospital's policies in advance so you can be realistic in your expectations.

☐ Keep reading, listening and learning about breastfeeding. You will become a valuable resource not only to your baby but to other breastfeeding mothers in the future.

CHAPTER 2

UNDERSTAND HOW THE MILK FACTORY WORKS

BREASTFEEDING DOESN'T HAVE TO SUCK if you understand the structure, manufacture and release of milk from the breast. By appreciating the inner workings of the 'milk factory', you will identify and solve problems faster and be more confident when breastfeeding.

LEARN THE BREAST BASICS

Most people can't remember very much about their anatomy from 10th Grade biology or their (embarrassing) health classes. Therefore it is not surprising that most of us know little about the female breast – especially as it is glamorized for its role in sex instead of feeding our children.

I find it ironic that many women want larger breasts so partners will find them more attractive. This attractiveness is linked to the breast in a very functional way. The partner's primal brain associates larger breasted women with the ability to make more milk and therefore have a better chance of keeping their offspring alive - so a more desirable mate. Subconsciously, partners understand the importance of breastfeeding!

Having a basic understanding of the anatomy and physiology of the breast and the process it goes through to create breastmilk helps women appreciate the process, understand how their bodies work and ultimately breastfeed better and longer.

I often compare breastmilk production to a *factory* that has two manufacturing units running at the same time. Like two breasts, the units work together in harmony. And like the ducts, alveoli and lobules, the assembly line that connects the product to the outside world occasionally has a hitch and needs help to get back on track. Expert mechanics – in the form of lactation consultants - are often called in to assist when a worker encounters something unusual.

The end product is the priceless milk. Consumer demand from the baby can be unpredictable and unrelenting! The logistics of manufacturing the milk and latching the baby to the breast for delivery can often be the hardest part. Let's start to understand some key information that can make or break your ability to run your own breastmilk operation efficiently.

THINK OF THE BREAST LIKE TREE BRANCHES

The internal anatomy of a breast is probably most comparable to the branches of a tree immersed in a bowl of fat and tissue with the main stalks terminating in the nipple! It is not wholly necessary to understand the intricate anatomy of the breast but knowing a few key facts can be useful knowledge.

The breast is shaped and cushioned by intraglandular fat (fatty tissue). That same fatty tissue is intertwined with glandular tissue that makes and stores milk. Inside the glandular tissue is milk making glands called alveoli which I compare to leaves. According to research performed by the University of Western Australia in 2006, the ratio of intraglandular fat and glandular tissue varies greatly between women and it is the amount of glandular tissue that determines the ability to make milk. That is why a small breasted woman (with a lot of glandular tissue and little fat tissue) may make a lot more milk than her larger breasted friend who has a lot of fat tissue and less glandular tissue. The moral of the paragraph is that you shouldn't assume you will struggle to make milk just because you were a 32 B cup. Conversely, don't assume that a 42 DDD will make gallons.

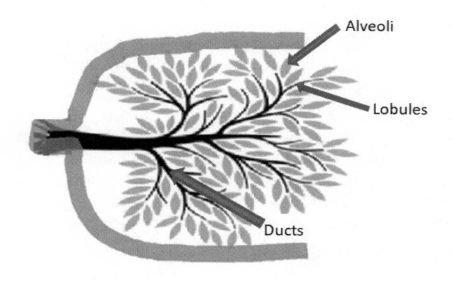

Ducts, Lobules and Alveoli

More than half of the glandular tissue is located within a 1 inch (30mm) radius from the base of the nipple and the ducts are fairly close to the skin's surface. Therefore **if you are supporting the breast with one hand, it is probably best to keep the hand close to your chest in a C shape against your rib cage**. If you inadvertently put pressure on the ducts and tissue in the front part of the breast, you could restrict milk flow. This, in turn, could lead to a plugged duct or blockage which could cause engorgement (a buildup of milk).

After being manufactured in the alveoli, the milk is sent down small branches (called lobules) to larger ones (called ducts). The 20+ ducts join on to the main trunk (referred to as a lobe). The lobe then directs the milk into a small spindle shaped reservoir where drops collect in a small pool.

When the baby draws milk out of the breast, it is initially being pulled out of the reservoir through thin *roots* (called lactiferous tubules) that terminate on the surface of the nipple and large brown circular areola. The end of the tubule is called a **nipple pore**. The baby needs to latch on to as many roots and bumps (nipple pores) as possible when feeding. The average woman has an average of 9 nipple pore openings although the range is 4-18.

Little bumps (called Montgomery Glands or Tubercles) on the areola are more prominent when pregnant and breastfeeding. Their job is to secrete an almost invisible lubricant that protects the sensitive brown skin. Similar to the sebaceous glands on your scalp, this lubricant keeps the area supple and moisturized – hence why **lanolin is not needed unless you have a cracked, scabbed or bleeding nipple**.

Before beginning a feed, it is useful to gently massage the breast to help *awaken* the alveoli and all the connecting ducts. It also helps milk start to flow into the ducts. Massaging closer to the chest wall can stimulate alveoli deeper in the breast. Breast pumps are good at emptying the front part of the breast but using hands when *combo pumping* (see pg. 170) gets to the milk further back in the breast.

WHAT DO A NIPPLE AND PENIS HAVE IN COMMON?

As a woman, you have probably realized that the nipple has one thing in common with the penis: it is made up of erectile tissue! The nipple is sensitive to stimulation and needs to be *aroused* in order to be able to evert (if inverted) and *stretch* well. The baby's suck causes that nipple arousal. In turn, **two hormones** kick start each breastfeeding journey as a result of that arousal.

The first hormone, called **prolactin**, signals the breast to start and continue milk production. Prolactin has a tranquilizing effect and mothers often report a yearning for their baby when prolactin is produced. Allowing the baby to feed on demand in the early weeks is the best way to keep prolactin levels high.

The second hormone needed for breastfeeding is **oxytocin**. In breastfeeding, oxytocin secretion 'turns on the tap' and allows milk to flow out. The start of milk flow is known as the ***Let Down Reflex*** (aka milk ejection reflex) and is stimulated when the baby latches onto the breast or the breast senses suction from a pump or other suction device. Many women feel let down as a *tingling sensation* on both sides. A fast letdown can initially be painful because milk is coming down the ducts quickly and stretching them a bit– sort of like opening the floodgates causes the riverbanks to swell initially. Let down occurs an average of *2.5 times per feed*, not just at the beginning of a feed. It can take several minutes for this reflex to completely activate.

If let down is slow, the hungry baby sucks faster until the milk starts to flow. Once the *tap is turned on*, the baby's sucking slows down. Some women feel an incredible thirst when they let down – it is referred to as the ***unquenchable thirst of let down***.

After breastfeeding is established, let down becomes a conditioned reflex - meaning that certain other situations can cause it to flow – like hearing a baby cry or seeing a photo of the baby. Wearing breast pads has stopped many embarrassing leakages through the mother's blouse when her let down is stimulated by another child or situation. I also forewarn women that the oxytocin produced during sexual arousal may also make her leak. Be prepared to drip some droplets of milk onto your partner's body right before orgasm!

PUMP THE BIG O AND AVOID THE BAD A

Besides being responsible for let down, oxytocin has many other amazing qualities. In labor, oxytocin is the naturally made wonder drug that causes contractions and keeps labor going. It is also the hormone of orgasm (hence why I really call it the BIG O), bonding, nurturing and falling in love. If a woman's natural oxytocin levels subside in labor (due to an epidural or lack of pelvic floor pressure from poor positions), care providers give her Pitocin (man-made oxytocin) through an IV to get labor going again.

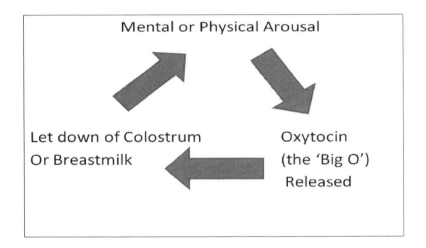

The Let Down Loop

The enemy of oxytocin is the 'Bad A' (Adrenaline). Adrenaline is a broad term for hormones that have a negative impact and cause stress. The Bad A can knock out the Big O with ease. That is why lovemaking can come to a sudden halt if one of the partners gets angry. That same Bad A can slow down or halt her let down in breastfeeding if the mother feels upset, stressed or angry.

Think carefully about where you will breastfeed and who you will have in the room with you. If a well-meaning relative makes negative comments about the mother's ability to breastfeed when she is trying to let down, *the tap may not turn on*. I always ask partners to be the breastfeeding **bouncer** in the early days – and get those well-intentioned people doing something else like food prep, cleaning, or running errands.

When I ask mothers who struggled with breastfeeding what the situation was like when they tried to feed, they often describe being with a well-meaning relative who said things like "Are you sure the latch is right?" or asked "Is the baby getting enough?". These comments were enough to cause adrenaline to pump in the weary mother which then stopped her oxytocin which then caused her NOT to let down very well.

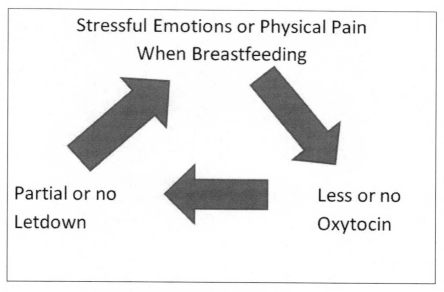

Stressful Emotions or Physical Pain When Breastfeeding

Partial or no Letdown

Less or no Oxytocin

The Effect of Stress on Breastfeeding

HEARD OF LIQUID GOLD?

In the first few days and weeks of having a new baby, what comes out of the breast will change in both **color and quantity**. The breast factory starts producing gold colored milk called **colostrum** (*nicknamed liquid gold*) around 14-16 weeks of pregnancy and this is the **first stage** of milk production. Colostrum is thicker milk with more condensed fat and protein than the more mature milk that develops after the first few days or week. That thicker colostrum is useful for the baby's tiny newborn stomach which is, on average, the size of a walnut. On Day 1, a newborn's stomach cannot stretch so overfeeding by bottle results in spitting up the excess.

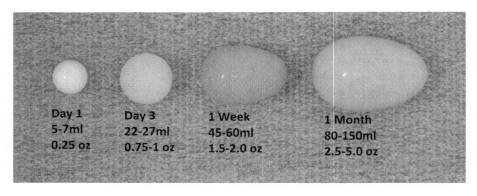

Average stomach sizes of a baby

Unlike breastfeeding, you can over feed a baby from a bottle as early as Day 2. The baby's stomach can stretch to hold more than the capacity shown above. Overfeeding starts to set up poor eating habits early. Just like the recommendation for adults, it is advised that babies eat little and often rather than large meals that cause the stomach to stretch.

While the baby is receiving colostrum, his or her diapers will probably contain meconium (dark colored molasses looking bowel movement). As the milk in the breast changes in color, quantity and consistency, meconium gives way to a lighter (spinach looking) bowel movement around day 2-4. By day 5, you should expect yellow mustard colored diapers full of both 'poop you can scoop' and stained mustard color wetness.

DOES MILK REALLY *COME IN?*

Eventually colostrum will be replaced by transitional milk. This **second part** of the breastfeeding process (lactogenesis II) usually happens somewhere between day 2-4 (but can be longer depending on birth factors) after the baby's birth and is referred to as *milk 'coming in'*. Blood flow inside the breast increases and the milk dilutes and increases in volume. During this changeover, some (but not all) women get *engorged (swollen)* hot breasts that benefit from cool packs and a little bit of hand expressing or hand-pumping before the baby feeds to relieve pressure. I compare it to going from manufacturing ice cream to manufacturing 2% fat milk.

This second stage of milk *coming in* is a CRITICAL time for breastfeeding because it is often when the baby is losing weight and fussy. The pressure is now on from the baby and the pediatrician for the mother's body to start milk production. In the mean-time, the mother is recovering from the birth and if her milk doesn't come in on time, she may readily consider giving up, supplementing with artificial baby milk or both.

In Chapter Three, we will discover some of the causes of a *delay in milk coming in* and in Chapter Nine we will learn how **early hand expressing and skin to skin contact ('skin to skin to bring milk in') can help get a mother over that hump.** Just remember that there is always something in the breast to feed the baby but *sometimes* giving the baby an ounce of artificial baby milk can help the baby through a crunch and **increase** the chance of breastfeeding success instead of failure.

HIT THE HINDMILK

The third and final part of the milk making process (lactogenesis III) is when the milk is established and maintained – usually around baby's day of life eight to ten. Milk will look light white and thin – a bit like cow's milk.

If you pump milk into a container, you will see it separate. The thinner lighter milk on the top has less fat and is referred to as **foremilk** and the milk with more fat that sinks to the bottom is called **hindmilk**. Think of the difference between milk and cream – both are milk but cream has more fat in it. It is important for a baby to feed long enough to get to the milk with a higher fat content **(pg. 64)**. A baby being exclusively fed breastmilk will have yellow bowel movements.

Sometimes *milk changes color (pg. 171)* depending on the baby's needs or the mother's diet. It may go a deeper yellow if the baby is ill as the mother's body increases antibodies and other naturally produced *medications* in her breastmilk.

FILL ME UP BUTTERCUP

One more thing to know about the breast is that if it is completely emptied, it completely refills – hence why cows that are milked daily produce milk for years. However if the breast is only partially emptied, a protein is created that allows only partial refilling. In lactation circles, this protein is referred to as the **Fil Factor**. This is why it is important to empty a breast thoroughly on a feed rather than switching to the other breast and giving the baby the same amount from each.

In **Chapter 5**, we will talk more about how to tell the baby is hungry, how often to feed and for how long.

SUMMARY:

☐ The breast is made up of a complex system of alveoli, lobules, ducts, and pores. Women all have a similar breast anatomy but some have more fatty tissue than others. Breast size is not always a good indicator of a woman's ability to breastfeed.

☐ The tubules terminate in the nipple. Montgomery glands are little bumps on the surface of the areola that secrete an oily substance to help lubricate and protect the surface of the skin.

☐ The nipple is aroused when the baby sucks on it. This arousal causes prolactin to turn on production and oxytocin to turn on the tap.

☐ If the woman is stressed when she is feeding, she may let down less or not at all because stress hormones reduce or stop oxytocin release.

☐ The process of making milk is called lactogenesis and is broken down into three stages. The first stage is the production of colostrum (16th week of pregnancy to 3 days after birth). Stage II (referred to as milk coming in) occurs somewhere between day 2-8 when the colostrum thins out and increases in volume. Stage III happens around day of life 8-10 when the milk is established and maintained.

☐ The color of the baby's bowel movements will change in color and consistency as the mother's milk supply moves through the three stages.

☐ It is important to completely empty one breast during a feed so that it fills up completely. If a breast is only partially depleted, it will not fully refill.

CHAPTER 3

REALIZE HOW LABOR & DELIVERY CAN AFFECT BREASTFEEDING (PARTNER*)

BREASTFEEDING DOESN'T HAVE TO SUCK if you understand how labor medications and procedures (Pitocin®, Syntocin®, fentanyl in an epidural, IV hydration) and postpartum solutions (immediate weighing and bathing, birth control pills, Benadryl® for itching, etc.) may impact breastfeeding and how to overcome roadblocks in the first several days postpartum.

It seems hard to believe, but once the baby is born, pregnancy and labor are quickly forgotten. As the mother begins breastfeeding, her labor experience could hamper or even sabotage her milk supply and cause her to begin doubting her ability to breastfeed. By knowing potential problems in advance, the mother can carry on with confidence and make educated decisions. In addition, getting help from a lactation consultant in those first few days can make a real difference.

UNDERSTANDING THE EFFECTS OF IV HYDRATION

In my childbirth class we often discuss labor interventions – those actions taken to improve a situation. When a woman is admitted to the labor unit, one of the first interventions that will be offered (and in many hospitals insisted upon) is an intravenous (IV) drip of saline, Ringer's Lactate or a dextrose solution through a vein on her hand or arm. The IV fluids are used to keep the mother hydrated and the total amount of fluid received in labor is referred to as the **fluid load** (measured in mL per hour).

Good hydration is really important in labor because it *keeps labor moving*. (Imagine running a nine hour race without being able to have sips or gulps of water along the way – you'd probably slow down or stop too). An IV for hydration is definitely an action taken to improve labor **(although hydrating via a water bottle for as long as possible should also be an option in many cases)**.

A woman who requests an **epidural** will have a ***mandatory IV*** of fluids to help maintain her blood pressure (which occasionally drops with an epidural). The epidural will ***not*** normally be sited until she has received *at least* 1000 mL of hydration. A woman who is being **induced with Pitocin or having an emergency or scheduled C-Section** will also have an IV drip for hydration usually from the time she is admitted. Most women who are induced or have a C-Section will receive anywhere between 1000-5000mL of fluid during the labor.

A large fluid load (**>2500ml**) can lead to the mother retaining water (peripheral edema). Water retention is not normally a problem for the mother because her body releases it over the next few days after birth through urination. However a large fluid load can cause three distinct breastfeeding issues.

First, **the baby's recorded weight at birth may be inflated** by that same water retention. Since all future weight gain (or loss) will be measured against that first number, accuracy is important. Most studies indicate that the true birth weight is most accurate somewhere at the **24 hour mark** – after the baby's first feed but also after the baby has released the excess fluid from the mother's IV through the diaper. A useful suggestion is to *"wait on the weight"* – ask to have the baby (re)*weighed 12 to 24 hours after birth* to obtain a true birthweight. That time lapse allows the baby to shed most of the excess water through their diaper, allows several colostrum feeds and gives a much better starting point from which to measure all future weight gain or loss. If the baby has more than one wet diaper in the first 24 hours, they are probably shedding excess fluid from the mother's IV.

Second, *third spacing fluid retention (excess fluid gathering in anything that hangs down in the extra cellular 'third space')* in the breast can cause inverted nipples and make latching a newborn particularly difficult. I've taken the odd phone call from a woman who was struggling to latch her newborn AND confused her waterlogged breast with a milk-engorged breast. In order to work out the difference, feel the firmness of the breast and examine the nipple. A milk-engorged breast feels similar to the firmness of your wrist and should not affect the nipple. Swelling of the breast with excess fluids feels similar to the firmness of the fleshy part of your arm and can cause the nipple to get pulled inward.

If you suspect your breast is swollen with excess fluids and/or the nipple is pulled inward, try a technique called Reverse Pressure Softening (pg. 77-78) to make it easier for the baby to latch on to a water laden breast. Also know that a woman who has had a big fluid load *may not engorge with milk at all* – but she will have milk in the breast eventually.

Finally, a large fluid load can create a **delay in milk diluting and increasing in volume ('coming in').** Remember from Chapter 2 that milk is expected to flood (engorge) the breast around **day 2-4**. A large fluid load can thin out colostrum, reduce or negate engorgement AND delay transitional milk *coming in for several days –resulting in a very hungry baby.*

LIFECYCLE OF BREaStFEEDInG FaiLURE

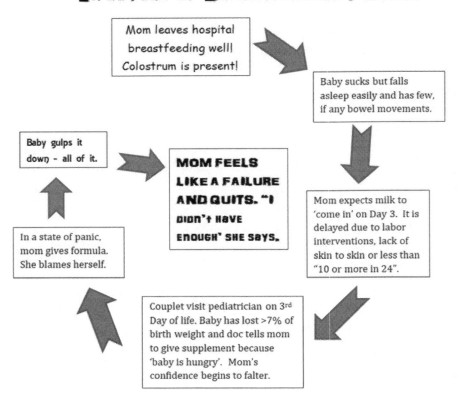

Mom leaves hospital breastfeeding well! Colostrum is present!

Baby sucks but falls asleep easily and has few, if any bowel movements.

Baby gulps it down - all of it.

MOM FEELS LIKE A FAILURE AND QUITS. "I DIDN't HaVE ENOUGH' SHE SayS.

Mom expects milk to 'come in' on Day 3. It is delayed due to labor interventions, lack of skin to skin or less than "10 or more in 24".

In a state of panic, mom gives formula. She blames herself.

Couplet visit pediatrician on 3rd Day of life. Baby has lost >7% of birth weight and doc tells mom to give supplement because 'baby is hungry'. Mom's confidence begins to falter.

This tends to occur after the mother has arrived home (without professional breastfeeding support) and the baby wants to load up on calories over a short period of time (called cluster feeding). *With a cranky baby and no sign of milk, the mother starts to blame her body for not functioning correctly, doubt her own abilities to produce, become anxious and jack-in breastfeeding before it really got started – all because of a well-intentioned intervention in labor!*

In order to combat the effects of over-hydration messing with the milk supply and transition, here are a few things you can do to get the milk rolling. **Continuous skin to skin time** with the baby (and allowing the baby to suck, suck, suck) in the first several days is the first line of defense for helping the breast to *manufacture milk*. My lactation instructor used to compare intensely long periods of sucking on day 2-3 as 'putting in an order at a restaurant' and then waiting a day or two for it to arrive. *My mantra is "Skin to skin to bring milk in".*

Hand expressing colostrum - especially in the first 48 hours after birth - is another wise way to combat milk coming in slowly; it can be stored and fed to the baby if needed (see Chapter 9) in many ways besides a bottle. Finally, **supplementing with a few ounces of artificial baby milk/formula or banked breastmilk** may seem counterproductive to breastfeeding but it can solve the immediate problem while the mother's body equalizes and in many cases can pave the way for a successful breastfeeding relationship instead of destroying it.

PITOCIN'S DOUBLE WHAMMY

As you just read, women receiving Pitocin® (*synthetic oxytocin*) to induce labor or help get stalled contractions revving again will have an **IV for hydration** which can cause a delay in milk manufacture. In addition, the *Pitocin ®itself* gives researchers cause for concern in breastfeeding because use of 'Pit' is also associated with reduced sucking in the first two hours after birth as well as delayed onset of milk production/milk coming in.

Naturally produced oxytocin crosses the blood-brain barrier and helps promote bonding, nurturing, milk creation, etc. Man-made Pitocin®

does cause regular contractions but does not cause those other wonderful qualities that the naturally produced oxytocin does. Therefore a prolonged IV for hydration *and* the use of 'Pit' creates a double whammy for a possible delay in the first few feeds being successful and a delay in milk flooding the breast on day 2-8. The same fixes for fluid overload should be used for the effect of Pitocin (continuous skin to skin, hand expression and, if necessary, an ounce or two of formula to get you over the hump).

WATCH OUT FOR OPIOIDS IN PAIN MEDS

More than 75% of women will request pain medication in labor – usually either a *narcotic* (like Morphine, Stadol, Fentanyl, Nubain or Demerol) or an *epidural* (containing Fentanyl). Pain medication in labor can be a *fabulous choice for many reasons* but studies suggest the opioids in the pain medications can be the first hurdle to successful breastfeeding. It would appear that the longer the woman has been under the influence of the opioid or epidural, the greater the potential impact on breastfeeding. If a woman has an epidural for greater than five hours (with a >2500ml fluid load), **it is likely that she won't get engorged at all.**

Some of the noted side effects of opioids in labor that may affect breastfeeding include breathing problems, decreased alertness, weak suck/poor latch, delay in mother's milk *'coming in'* and lack of skin to skin in the first few hours or days after birth. The best suggestion – if possible – is to skip narcotics in labor and have an epidural as late as one can manage (>5 cm+) to reduce or avoid previously mentioned problems and *employ the same fixes* for fluid overload and Pitocin's double whammy.

> *Pain medications are your choice during labor. Realize that if your milk is delayed coming in, it is not your fault and you are doing nothing wrong!*

BABY OR MAMA TRAUMA?

Recently I attended a lecture given by a chiropractor specializing in pediatrics. She highlighted how care providers often assist babies out of their mother's bodies (in both vaginal and C-Section births) with one hand on the baby's jaw and the other hand on the back of the skull. Gentle pulling probably does not harm but many times the pulling can be very aggressive and affect the baby's neck.

Over half of the patients that the chiropractor treated were under a year old and had symptoms such as colic, reflux, torticollis (baby's head persistently turned to one side) and plagiocephaly (flat or misshapen head). Many babies whose heads are pulled aggressively during delivery struggle to open their mouths wide and this, in turn, affects latch. If your baby experienced a rough delivery, consider consulting with a chiropractor who is a member of the International Chiropractic Pediatric Association or a cranial osteopath.

Another type of birth trauma can affect the mother and her ability to breastfeed. Although **rare**, there is a condition called **Sheehan's Syndrome** which is a form of shock brought on by *severe* bleeding when the placenta is delivered in the third and final stage of labor. The bleeding causes the mother's blood pressure to drop so low that blood fails to circulate to her pituitary gland and some or all of the cells in that gland stop working permanently. Her breasts remain soft and she may not be able to produce milk. Sadly, this is a permanent malfunction and may mean she is completely unable to breastfeed.

GET SKIN TO SKIN AS MUCH AS POSSIBLE

It wasn't that long ago that newly born babies cords were cut immediately so they could be carted off to a *warmer* to be assessed, weighed, dried and cleaned before being diapered, wrapped up and handed back to the mother with no skin to skin contact. Hospitals that are certified members of the **Baby Friendly Hospital Initiative** (BFHI) strive to assess the baby while he/she is lying on their mother and promote skin to skin contact and breastfeeding in the first 60 minutes after the birth before moving everyone to the postpartum unit. The postpartum nurses are also skilled in hand expression. Is your hospital part of the Baby Friendly Hospital Initiative?

Lack of skin to skin contact in the first few days of life is one of the best ways to cause ***breastfeeding failure***. Putting the baby's skin against the mother's skin immediately after the baby is born helps to regulate the baby's body temperature, stabilize breathing, increase glucose levels, reduce both the baby and mother's stress hormones, regulate blood pressure and decrease crying. You cannot show me one machine that can do all that skin to skin can do!

Most importantly, that first hour of skin to skin (known as the **Golden Hour**) contact should be a ***minimum*** of 60 minutes. The more skin to skin contact a baby receives in the first two weeks, the more likely that a great breastfeeding relationship will be established.

After your baby is born, watch him to see if he exhibits the **nine newborn behaviors** (intense crying just after birth, relaxing, awakening, active phase, crawling/pushing, resting at the nipple, suckling and sleeping) in the golden hour(s). There is a very good video clip (3.11 min) on youtube.com called *Important Findings Published About Common Labor Medications and Breastfeeding Success* (Healthy Children Project, 2015) that shows the nine behaviors and discusses how medications in labor can affect breastfeeding.

If you watch any of the '*Breast Crawl*' video clips online, you will see an alert baby (whose mother has had very few interventions) maneuver himself to the mother's breast through smell, salivate when he gets near and eventually attach his tiny mouth onto the nipple completely unaided. Babies are born wanting to breastfeed but well-intentioned interventions can upset this process.

THINK THROUGH POSTNATAL DECISIONS

Depending on the delivery, a mother usually leaves the hospital in 24-48 hours. During the short time in the postpartum unit, beware of some of the well-intended practices and medications that may upset early milk production.

Postpartum nurses are normally happy to demonstrate or assist in the **baby's first bath**. Current research suggests waiting a minimum of anywhere from **12-24 hours to bathe the baby**. This allows any protective vernix (white cheesy looking substance) still visible on the baby's skin to be absorbed - which in turn helps to protect the baby from a number of nasty pathogens that lurk in hospitals. It is also important that the *baby's hands are not washed for the first 12 (or more) hours because the smell of amniotic fluid on the hands is the same smell given off by the mother's breast*. This smell is what guides him or her to sniff out the trail of the nipple.

Benadryl (Diphenhydramine) is used in labor to help reduce itching from an epidural. It is also the magic cure to reduce swelling in a swollen cervix ('lip'). Using this drug on the laboring or postnatal women is done with the best of intent for good reason. However the reference database Lactmed states *"Larger doses or more prolonged use may cause effects in the infant or decrease the milk supply, particularly in combination with a sympathomimetic such as pseudoephedrine before lactation is well established"*.

While many care providers feel that a single small dose of Benadryl will not affect colostrum or the flooding of the breast in stage 2, there is very little research on the topic. It may be better to err on the side of caution and ask what other alternatives could be used.

Women who have a Cesarean Section or a severe tear will be offered medication to help with the surgery pain. T3 (a short name for Tylenol with Codeine) and Oxycodone are drugs **commonly** given for pain but neither is recommended if the mother is breastfeeding. Hospitals are slowly changing but it is always worth asking or plugging in the name of the drug on the **National Lactmed database (https://www.toxnet.nlm.nih.gov)** to see what effect a drug will have on breastfeeding.

As you leave the hospital, it is not uncommon for well-meaning care providers to discuss birth control with the mother since many women will resume sex before their six week check. Birth control pills that contain **estrogen can reduce or halt a milk supply.** The World Health Organization and many manufacturers' recommendations suggest that ANY birth control that releases anything into the body that could alter hormone production be avoided for the **first six weeks** of breastfeeding. Preferred alternatives include intrauterine devices (IUDs), progestin-only oral contraceptives (mini pill) or progestin-only implants (ex. Norplant) or condoms! While you would think every care provider would know the effect estrogen can have on a milk supply, I have come across several care providers who prescribed birth control pills containing estrogen to a breastfeeding mother without warning her.

> **TIP**: Breastmilk does an amazing job of giving the baby most every nutrient that they need. However most all babies are born with a shortage of **Vitamin D** and the American Academy of Pediatrics recommend giving the baby 400 IU (international units) of liquid Vitamin D per day. Be sure to read the instructions and use the dropper provided. Many women find it easier putting the droplet of Vitamin D on their nipple right before the first feed of the day.

In Chapter 9 we will discuss things that can decrease a supply and also milk-increasing remedies (galactagogues) that can help *increase a supply*. Remember to ask your care providers if they are administering or prescribing anything that could have a possible impact on your milk supply.

SUMMARY:

☐A large intravenous (IV) fluid load (>2500 cc) in labor can cause a delay in milk diluting and increasing in volume (aka 'coming in'), inflate the baby's true birth weight and cause third spacing fluid retention. Fluid retention in the breast makes latching more difficult and is often confused with engorgement.

☐Use of Pitocin (synthetic oxytocin) during labor has been shown to reduce sucking in the first two hours after birth and reduce the overall success of long term breastfeeding.

☐Recording the baby's weight at birth is traditional but is not necessarily accurate if the mother has had a large fluid load. Weighing the baby several hours after the first feed (12-24 hours) is likely to give you a more realistic birthweight from which to compare future growth.

☐The *breastfeeding cycle of failure occurs* when the milk is slow to change from colostrum to transitional milk – usually due to labor drugs or interventions. The mother's breastfeeding confidence can easily be shattered if she does not think her body is capable of making enough.

☐Pain medications containing fentanyl (most epidurals) can delay or reduce engorgement and the transition from colostrum to transitional milk ('coming in'). The nine newborn behaviors may also be impaired by Fentanyl and Pitocin.

☐Birth trauma to either the baby or the mother can affect

breastfeeding. Aggressive delivery of the baby (by pulling on the head) can lead to neck issues. Severe bleeding in 3rd stage may cause the inability to produce milk.

☐ Skin to skin contact between the baby and the mother in the first two weeks is one of the best ways to establish successful breastfeeding. The golden hour should be a *minimum* of sixty minutes.

☐ During and after birth, medications like Benadryl (for epidural itching or cervical swelling), T3 (Tylenol with codeine) for pain or birth control containing estrogen could inhibit a fragile milk supply. Always ask care providers or pharmacists what affect any drugs can have on breastfeeding.

☐ Read the label on any medications that you take and if in doubt about their effect on breastfeeding or milk supply, refer to the website Lactmed **(https://www.toxnet.nlm.nih.gov**) to assess safety.

☐ A woman who labors without an epidural (or a very late epidural) and delivers vaginally is less likely, if at all, to suffer from a delay in milk coming in, an inflated birthweight or fluid retention causing latching problems.

JESSICA'S STORY – A SWOLLEN START

My birth plan was somewhat of a unique situation because I knew an epidural was not possible. A few years before my pregnancy, I had an emergency spinal fusion which meant my birth would be either an un-medicated (no epidural) vaginal birth or a cesarean under general anesthesia where I was knocked out completely. Happily for me, I was able to find supportive care with providers that would allow me the most possible freedom of choice.

Due to some pregnancy complications, my labor was started with an emergency induction using Cytotec (a drug that ripens the uterus and often kick starts contractions) in pill form. I was hydrated with an IV fluid drip starting on a Friday night. The Cytotec worked really well and I never needed Pitocin but I did labor long and hard. After working through contractions with a hyper stimulated uterus for 24 hours, I felt I could no longer go on this way and 'called it' – I wanted to move to cesarean. The staff honored my choice, moved me to the operating room and prepped me for surgery.

Although the baby was born quickly, I had considerable blood loss which led to me receive even more IV fluids to avoid a transfusion. I probably had at least 4000 cc (1 gallon) of lactated ringers in total. Thankfully the bleeding eventually stopped and I woke up after recovery ready to meet my baby and breastfeed!

My little girl weighed 8lbs 15 oz. and seemed in good health. ***However I noticed that I looked very different.*** Although I was no longer pregnant, I had swollen hands, swelling in my face and breasts so swollen that my once protruding nipples had gone flat. This was not my anatomy! I had no idea that retaining all that fluid could cause your breasts to swell. I tried so hard to get her to latch on to my stretched flat nipple. At the nurse's suggestion I tried a nipple shield but that did not help.

None of the nurses mentioned that the retained IV fluids were to blame so I blamed myself. I felt so awful for not being able to latch my baby! Nurses and lactation consultants repeatedly referred to my "flat nipples" as the problem, but I just kept thinking, "I don't have flat nipples". Over the next four days, I anxiously waited for my milk to come in. In the meantime, the baby was quickly losing weight – 15% in total. Although I was discharged, it was decided that the baby would be kept another night as we continued to try to get her to latch and bring my milk in.

Despite me being with her 24/7, FORMULA was ordered. I cried hysterically as soon as they brought the formula into the room. Even though she was finally able to latch to my breast, she was supplemented with expressed colostrum and FORMULA using a medicine cup. (I didn't want her getting used to a bottle as well!) In the end, she only received formula for 24 hours because my milk came in with a rush on the next night (Day 5). Once my milk came in, I never needed formula again.

It was about a week until I didn't feel swollen from the cesarean fluids anymore. Looking back on it, I had thought that using formula would signal an end to my breastfeeding relationship. In fact, it ended up being what saved it. We just finished breastfeeding after 2.5 years!

AUTHOR'S NOTE: Jessica's story demonstrates how necessary intervention during labor – in this case a heavy fluid load causing '3rd spacing' – can interfere with early breastfeeding success. It is a shame that the nurses did not suggest the **reverse pressure softening technique (pg. 78)** which may have allowed the baby to latch. Thankfully this warrior mother persevered and was able to establish breastfeeding. This story is also a reminder that supplementing with formula for clinical need can save a breastfeeding relationship instead of destroying it.

CHAPTER 4

SURVIVING THE FIRST 14 DAYS
(PARTNER*)

BREASTFEEDING DOESN'T HAVE TO SUCK *if you are prepared for the ups and downs of the early days, understand cluster feeds and appreciate the 'poop loop' in order to avoid the 'two week weakness' and give up.*

Most pregnant mothers have a hard time thinking about life after labor – I know I did. Labor lasts an *average of 13-20 hours* but the first two weeks of life with a newborn lasts *336 hours* - so preparation is key. This chapter discusses the vital first two weeks after the baby is born, how to get breastfeeding off to a great start and how to maintain the momentum.

Once the baby is born (and assuming the baby is healthy), he or she is checked, weighed and measured and then put *skin to skin* with the mother. Most hospitals will weigh and measure the baby in the first hour of birth and assess the baby (APGAR scoring) while he/she is lying on the mother's abdomen. The placenta is also delivered and the mother is cleaned up with a warm sponge bath. Perineal repair, if necessary, is usually done immediately after the birth too.

Finally you, your partner and the baby are given time to get to know each other, bond *and hopefully feed the baby* during the *golden hour (60+ minutes after the baby is born)*. After that, you are wheeled out of Labor & Delivery and into the postpartum unit. Then what?

Usually the mother and partner want to tell everyone the joyous news and get some rest. The early days of having a new baby are usually filled with steep learning curves and getting used to the *new normal*. The first two weeks of breastfeeding are often the hardest - hence why I refer to that time period as the *'two week weakness'*. Roughly 81% of women attempt to breastfeed but 15% give up before being discharged and only 32% of women reach their goal. This chapter is full of tips for surviving those first two weeks and getting breastfeeding off to the best possible start.

FEED DURING THE GOLDEN HOUR

This first hour together with the baby is called the *Golden Hour* because it is expected (or at least hoped) that the baby will be alert enough to search out the breast and latch for his or her first feed of *golden colored colostrum*. As mentioned in Chapter 3, newborns that have *no* medications in their system are more likely to be alert and exhibit the nine basic newborn behaviors that lead to latching and feeding in that first hour. A big feed is often followed by a big sleep - sort of like going to a wild party where you stay up late and then come home to sleep it off!

However, if your baby is not particularly alert, sleepy or keeps nodding off (for any number of reasons), that first feed may take far longer to initiate. In the semi reclining position (pg. 91) and with the baby skin to skin, try latching the baby every ten minutes or so until you are successful. Get help if you are struggling. The breasts are ready to feed the baby.

HAND EXPRESS IN THE EARLY HOURS & DAYS

Regardless of whether the baby manages a good feed in that first hour or not, it is also really important – **IF YOU CAN MANAGE IT - to** *hand express* (remove from the breast with your own two hands) colostrum in the first hour after birth. Research indicates that **both** a feed AND *hand expressing another teaspoon* during the golden hour *is* the **best way to stimulate a super supply**. In an important 2012 study, women hand expressing a teaspoon of colostrum within the first hour after birth had more mature milk transitioning into the breast (milk 'coming in') faster and up to a 130% increase in milk supply at the six week mark.

Hand expressing can be daunting (especially after a mentally and physically exhausting labor) but colostrum is **not** easily removed from the breast with an electric pump. (For directions on hand expressing technique, see pg. 165-166). Your postpartum nurse should also be able to help. You can catch those hand expressed drops in a sterile plastic medicine cup and feed that extra teaspoon of colostrum to the baby with a dropper (or ask the nurse to label and store in the refrigerator for later).

If you can't manage hand expressing in the first hour, try hand *expressing in the first few days after birth*. In that same 2012 study, women who hand expressed **six times per day in the first three days after birth increased their milk supply by 45% at the six week mark** compared to women who had hand expressed two or less times a day over the same postpartum time period. WOW!

Finally, if you were not able or do not want to hand express, do not *beat yourself up!* Many of you will be reading this after your return from the hospital and there are other ways to build a dependable supply (see Chapter 9).

LET THE BABY SUCK TO TRIGGER THE *POOP LOOP*

Babies are born with a few instinctive behaviors necessary for survival and finding the breast is probably the strongest one. The baby has a keen instinct to suck – especially in the first few days. This is like *requesting a drink from the tap and priming the pump*. It can take a lot of priming before the tap actually releases much more than foam.

It is the same with the breast. Colostrum in the breast is enough for the baby in the first few days but sucking a lot primes the breast to produce a higher volume of milk a few days later that will satisfy him as he grows. Not only is the baby priming the pump; he is putting in his order for the next several rounds!

The other reason that the baby sucks a lot in the early days is to help *push out the meconium* (first poop). Babies are basically born full of meconium and sucking helps to stimulate his or her little body to force it out to the diaper. Expect the first few dirty diapers to look black and tar like.

I refer to this sucking cycle (sucking a lot, priming the pump & pushing out the meconium) as the *Poop Loop*. The baby sucks a lot to place the order for milk production, the milk is delivered a few days later and the sucking also helps the baby to rid their body of meconium poop.

FEED 10 OR MORE IN 24

Most breastfeeding advice will tell you to feed the baby eight or more times a day in the first week. It would appear that, while eight times a day is probably adequate, feeding the baby **ten or more times a day**

in those first four days almost guarantees that the baby will suck enough to bring in the mature milk, regain his/her birthweight and potentially avoid jaundice (pg. 142).

A feed takes as little as a few minutes or as long as the baby needs – some are slower and some are faster. *Aim for 15-25 minutes* on the first breast and 5-15 minutes on the second but do not time feeds or take the baby off the breast if they are still actively sucking. *Young babies often need only one breast at a feed*. Concentrate on taking the time to empty one breast completely as opposed to offering a little from each. *Emptying a breast may take 20 minutes or more.*

Feeding a baby 10 or more times in 24 hours means that you may be feeding a baby (*for example*) at 5am, 7.30am, 9.30am, Noon, 2pm, 4.30pm, 7pm, 9.30pm, 11pm and 2.30am before starting the day over again at 5am. It is A LOT of feeding but once the mature milk is 'in' and the baby is gaining weight, the baby will probably feed more efficiently each time and also less often as his or her stomach grows.

SURVIVE DAY OF LIFE 1-3

Those first three days of having a newborn are filled with highs and lows. First and foremost, the mother is recovering from the birth. This is easier for some mothers than others depending on the length of labor, her emotional experience, use of drugs and medications, and vaginal versus C-Section. She is also now expected to feed the baby 10+ times a day! Visitors are eager to see her and meet the new family member but equally the mother needs rest.

On **Day One** in the hospital, the baby may sleep for several hours (*birthday nap*) after the first feed. This is normal but the baby should still be offered the breast *8+ times in the first 24 hours*. I know that seems like a huge effort after labor but it is probably one of the easiest things you can do to fire up your milk supply in the days to come. I recall that my baby slept for six hours after birth and I had no idea that I'd missed two feeds.

<u>You will probably need to wake the baby and encourage him or her to feed</u> in those first 24+ hours. Rubbing the baby's back or feet and cooling them down a little can awaken their appetite. **If you just can't arouse the baby from sleep, hand express 20 drops from each breast when you would have fed in that first 24 hours.**

Day Two is usually the day you are discharged from the hospital. It is also often the day that the **baby wants to suck a lot** to *trigger the breast to bring in the higher volume of milk in the coming days*. This is an important day for skin to skin contact with the mother. Remember: **"Skin to skin to bring milk in"**!

Day Three is a crucial one. First of all, it is the day that most women return to the care provider for the baby's first checkup. It is also the day women are expecting their milk to 'come in' - any delay can make the mother feel like a failure. If the baby has lost >7% of his or her birthweight, it is also the day that the pediatrician will recommend, demand or force formula feeding on you (see *The Breastfeeding Lifecycle of Failure* on pg. 36). Just remember that formula can be a useful bridge to get you over the hump. The reason your milk is delayed is usually due to your labor experience. Breastfeed and use formula, donor milk or milk you expressed in the days beforehand until your milk is fully in.

> **TIP: Day three** after the birth is a crucial one. It is the first point at which many women give up – usually blaming themselves for not having enough milk. Hang in there, keep cluster feeding and remember: Skin to Skin to bring milk in!

Night three is also usually a challenge! This is the night when the mother may experience the baby **cluster feeding** for the first time – I call it the 'all you can eat buffet' night. That means that the baby may want to feed every hour for several hours as they **load up on calories**. Remember that if there is a delay in milk flooding the breast (for any of the reasons mentioned previously), you may have a fussy cranky baby on your hands. Hang on in there and keep the baby skin to skin as much as you can manage.

If you doubt that you have anything in the breast, try hand expressing or hand pumping (*pg. 166*) for a few minutes to convince yourself. You can feed those drops to the baby with a spoon, cup or dropper. **Remember** that let down can take a minute or more and that stress can stop it from happening. If you do have a *severe delay* in milk flooding the breast, you may consider supplementing with an ounce or two of artificial baby milk to get you over the hump. But ideally, 'breastmilk is bestmilk' because of the way it lines the baby's gut with healthy bacteria – especially in those crucial early days.

On the other hand, if you notice milk flooding the breast quickly, you may get engorged (swollen) breasts. This can make it hard for the baby to get a good mouthful of nipple and areola because the breast gets hard like a cantaloupe. In order to latch and attach the baby on to an engorged breast, hand express or use a manual pump to soften the breast to more of a water balloon consistency.

DON'T FREAK OUT AT THE 1ˢᵀ DOCTORS VISIT

Assuming all is stable, most mothers (and babies) will leave the hospital within 24-36 hours of birth. Before they leave, the baby's first appointment with the pediatrician will normally be scheduled – usually within a few days. At that first doctor's appointment, the baby will be weighed to assess weight gain or loss. Remember that the weight loss **'scare-o-meter'** starts ticking from birth so that is why I recommend weighing the baby again at the 12-24 hour mark to establish a true birthweight.

This first appointment can be very stressful for the mother. She often feels as if she is being graded for her first *parental report card*. Even though babies are expected to lose up to 10% of their birth weight, loss of more than 6% -7% on day 3 or 4 usually triggers the doctor into discussing, introducing or forcing formula milk. This can be hard for a new mother to process emotionally because it can make her feel like body has already failed her.

As a reminder from Chapter 3, remember that the drugs used in labor can affect (slow down) milk *coming in* and that the birthweight is most accurate at the 24 hour mark if she had an IV for fluids, induction with Pitocin® or an epidural containing fentanyl. If milk is not in yet, supplementing with pumped colostrum, donor milk or (if necessary) formula is a quick fix. But skin to skin, hand expressing a teaspoon after every feed and letting the baby suck (to trigger the poop loop) are also ways to help bring in the more mature milk.

As the baby and mother start to establish breastfeeding in those first few days, breastfeeding starts to get easier or sometimes much harder. If the baby is not latched deep enough, this is when nipple and areola damage often starts. We will talk about latch in great detail in Chapter Six but if you are starting to have damage when the baby feeds, get help when you go to the 1st Doctor's visit. If the doctor can't help you, ask to be referred to a lactation clinic or specialist as soon as possible. Sometimes a small change can make a big difference and it is often hard to spot the problem by yourself.

WORK AS A TEAM (DAY OF LIFE 3-7)

Usually the first week is a quiet time for everyone. You and the baby are getting used to being at home. If you have a partner, family member or friend helping you, make sure they are actually part of the team rather than trying to be the coach. Negative comments in these early days can really dent a woman's confidence. If you are too polite to say anything directly, either go to another (private) room to feed or ask them to do some shopping, cleaning or cooking for you. Early breastfeeding requires an adrenaline free environment to go well.

Day 3 to 7 is when the flood of milk usually begins to arrive and babies are getting slightly more efficient at removing milk from the breast. Babies have usually lost weight over the first three days and this is hopefully the beginning of eating enough to put that weight back on over the next week. Concentrate on feeding and taking care of the baby and yourself. Everything else can wait.

Most guidebooks will tell you to look for a certain number of wet and dirty diapers as your guide (see page 66) to the baby's healthy intake and that can be useful. But breastfed babies' diapers can be somewhat unpredictable in those first few weeks so look for consistent patterns rather than hitting a certain number of diapers every day. Following the *10 or more in 24* feeding rule is probably a better way to make sure the baby is getting enough rather than obsessing over diaper counts. What goes in must come out.

WATCH OUT FOR THE TWO WEEK WEAKNESS

After a week of having a quiet and often drowsy newborn, babies tend to become a bit more vocal in the second week. This is also the time when the partner may go back to work and the mother is left alone for the majority of the day to care for the baby. When you are recovering from a birth, feeding a baby ten times a day, sleep deprived and possibly highly emotional from baby blues, it is easy to quit breastfeeding. That is why I label the 2nd week as the 'Two Week Weakness'.

Getting out of the house can also be a challenge but one that is worth doing. My sister told me that every time she planned an outing and put a special outfit on her son, he routinely threw up minutes before they were due to leave! Find a breastfeeding support group or mother's circle to get some social interaction with other like-minded souls. In this second week, the mother's goals have not changed: **she should feed herself, feed her baby, have a shower and get as much rest as possible.**

At the 2nd Doctor's appointment, the pediatrician is expecting the baby to be gaining weight. If the baby weighs in well, the mother will come out of the doctor's office relieved and happy. But if the baby is still losing or gaining very slowly, the pediatrician will want the baby to be supplemented with artificial baby milk. This can dent a mother's confidence further and possibly convince her that she doesn't have enough or isn't efficient at making enough milk (see *Lifecycle of Breastfeeding Failure* – pg.36).

SUPPLEMENT IF NECESSARY

Supplementation - that is giving the baby a small amount of milk not from the breast – is a dirty word in many breastfeeding circles. Having said that, giving the baby extra milk (artificial formula milk, donor milk or Medolac) can be a clinically necessary short term move if there is a delay in milk flooding the breast, the baby sucks but does not swallow, weight loss is continuous or the mother's supply is truly low. It does not mean that the mother will dry up, be unable to breastfeed or has 'given in'.

Milk that has been expressed, dripped or pumped (see Chapter 12) earlier in the day can also be used to supplement the baby at the part of the day where the mother is most tired and her supply is thought to be lowest – often in the late afternoon or early evening. **You can also mix breastmilk and formula in the same bottle.**

HOLD ON TO YOUR BABY

Newborns take their time adjusting to the outside world of bright lights, loud noises and big smells. They are very sensitive to the new environment around them. All they really want is to be skin to skin against their mother's warm body, listening to her heartbeat, smelling her smell, feeling safe and feeding when hungry. A lot of visitors passing a newborn around can impact the new baby's behavior and breastfeeding success. When a new baby cries, it means he is either very hungry, in pain or scared. Often visitors feel that they should try to quiet the baby rather than giving him back to the Mother for some skin to skin and possible feeding opportunity.

In those first several weeks, hold on to your baby as much as you can. I know you have been pregnant for 40 or so weeks and it would be nice to have a vacation from carrying the baby. But the first 14 days are really important for setting up a great breastfeeding and sleeping relationship. Skin to skin doesn't wear thin in the early weeks.

SUMMARY:

☐In the first week of life, skin to skin and breastfeeding are probably the most important factors in keeping your baby healthy. Skin to skin in the first few minutes and hours after the baby is born is important to bond and hopefully stimulate the baby's desire to suck and feed.

☐Hand expressing a teaspoon of milk in the first hour improves milk supply dramatically. Expressing after a feed in the first few days is also extremely useful in building a supply.

☐Feed the baby at least eight times in 24 hours on **day one**.

☐Aim to feed the baby 10 or more times in 24 hours on day **two through seven** of life or until the baby has regained his or her birthweight.

☐Babies may suck a lot and cluster feed in the first few days or nights. This does not mean that you are not producing enough milk for them. Sucking initiates the *poop loop* that helps them bring milk into the breast and clear meconium from their own bodies.

☐ Cluster feeding is when a baby feeds a lot over a short period of time (2-6 hours) – often on night three. Behavior of this type is normal and is the baby loading up on calories. It is often followed by a big sleep and is probably the result of the first growth spurt.

☐ Day 3-7 can be particularly challenging if the breast engorges and the baby struggles to latch OR the mother's milk has a delay in flooding the breast. Hand pumping or expressing can be very useful in both cases.

☐ At the baby's first doctor visit, weight gain or loss will be assessed. Remember that the baby's true birth weight is usually most accurate around the 24 hour mark. Supplementing can be a useful short term fix in many circumstances.

☐ At Day 10-14, the pediatrician expects the baby to have regained their birthweight and start putting on roughly an ounce a day in the first month. This can put particular pressure on a mother whose milk was slow to flood the breast.

☐ Supplementing (giving a bit extra) with either pumped or collected breastmilk or formula can help fill up a baby when the mother's own milk supply is low. Once the mother's supply stabilizes, supplementing is not necessary.

WHAT WERE THE FIRST FEW DAYS LIKE?

FROM ANGELINA: The beginning is kind of a blur, lol. After being discharged from the hospital, I think we had only had one night home before I saw the pediatrician for a follow up appointment. I was glad to go back so soon because I had a million questions and concerns. I remember being really scared to leave the house so my mom drove and my husband and I sat in the back seat. My baby weighed 6lbs13oz and at that first appointment was down to 6lbs 2oz. The pediatrician was nervous about weight loss (11oz loss = 10%) and jaundice because the baby's bilirubin was still pretty high.

She said I needed to "get him eating more" and scheduled me to come back a couple days later to be weighed again. She talked about switching to formula if there wasn't a quick improvement. At that point, I asked to see a Lactation Consultant and they walked me over to one in the next department! The Consultant helped me tremendously with the latch. I went back a few days later and the baby was almost back to birth weight! Our latch improved a lot over the next few weeks although we went back to the Consultant to trouble shoot other things. My tip is to use all the support you can!

FROM JENNY: My baby George was born on a Wednesday and we were home by Thursday afternoon. I took him to urgent care on Friday though because he wasn't pooping and peeing enough and he looked yellow. I totally forgot his diaper bag so I had to run (more like waddle) to labor and delivery to ask for supplies. I was A MESS. The pediatrician we saw at urgent care actually gave me her cell phone number if I had questions and to check on test results.

We had George's first pediatrician visit scheduled for Saturday (Day 3). I was exhausted and scared. His numbers were better than they had been in Urgent Care but the doctor ordered us a bili blanket. The blanket didn't come and it was impossible to get the pediatrician on the phone. I ended up calling the Urgent Care doctor and she put a rush on the bili blanket. Slowly the jaundice cleared.

The baby's one month check-up was awful because it seemed so RUSHED. I had so many questions but I arrived late – scared and sleep deprived. I cried. I look back at that time and I think of how far I've come. I will definitely tell him that story when he gets older. I'm a first time mom and there are so many things I'm learning. Today I learned my stroller fits in the front seat. My trunk wouldn't open for some reason, he was crying and I had to get home. My tip is to improvise where necessary!

FROM KATHERINE: Day 3 was the worst. He was weighed and of course not gaining enough so I had to do the supplemental nursing system attached to my breast. I also was given some tips on a better latch. I felt like such a failure that I could not provide enough. With my 2nd baby, I showed up for my Day 3 appointment but my regular doc was out so I had to be seen by another doctor. They poked Bella's feet 2 times to get blood because she was jaundiced. They checked her length and weight. Then I want to see the Lactation Consultant and found out that everything the doctor told me about breastfeeding was wrong (when, how long, etc.). My tip is to get help from a Lactation Specialist as soon as possible. I was surprised about the misinformation I received!

FROM EMMANUELA - I cried a lot! I had a great birth but it was impossible to get any breastfeeding help on the phone quickly. It took 48-72 hours to get any response from a professional. My tip is to learn as much about breastfeeding as you can before the first latch!

AUTHOR'S NOTE: The early days of having a newborn can be rough. The mother is recovering from the birth and breastfeeding an infant! When we are upset it is not uncommon to get flustered, forget things and feel like a total failure. In a few weeks, you will look back and wonder how you managed. But you will!

CHAPTER 5

WORK OUT WHEN THE BABY IS HUNGRY & WHEN THE BABY HAS HAD ENOUGH (PARTNER*)

***BREASTFEEDING DOESN'T HAVE TO SUCK** if you can recognize when a baby is hungry and how long to feed on each breast. Waiting until a baby is 'hangry' (hungry and angry) makes latching more difficult. Overfeeding can lead to excessive weight gain.*

It is easy to figure out when my teenagers are hungry – they walk into the kitchen, root around in the refrigerator, open drawers, look in the pantry and weigh up the food options. They eat because they are hungry, bored or worried. It is also relatively easy to figure out when my kids are full: they slow down their eating, eventually putting down their knives and forks and leaving the table.

Babies are similar to teenagers: they have varying stages of hunger and can want to eat for different reasons. The hunger signs are sometimes less obvious with babies. It can also be harder to determine if he or she has 'had enough' since you can't measure how much they are taking out of the breast. With early weight gain so important, it is no surprise that we focus on what and how much our children are eating for the rest of their lives.

LOOK FOR THE FEEDING CUES

Most people experience pangs or pains when they are hungry. Babies are no different. The pain of hunger is actually caused by small stomach contractions caused by the hormone ghrelin. Babies feel those same pangs and signal they are hungry in many ways.

One of the early signs (cues) is **lip, tongue and mouth movement** – similar to the way we lick our lips or move our mouth and tongue around without realizing it. Another sign is **movement of the hands and feet**. When babies are very hungry, they often **clench their fists** and **curl their toes**. As the baby transfers milk from your breast to his or her stomach, they slowly unfold their hands and feet. A baby that is relaxed after a feed is a sure sign of one that has been fed well.

My favorite hunger sign is the **rooting reflex**. Similar to most mammals, a baby roots by opening his/her mouth and/or turning his/her head while searching for the breast - similar to the way a bird opens its beak waiting for regurgitated food to be dropped in. I love watching a baby root for a nipple on a non-lactating adult – it usually startles them into handing the baby back to the mother quickly.

Crying is a last resort plea for food. We probably rely on crying far more than we should as a feeding cue. It can be much harder to latch a crying, upset, hunger-panging baby rather than one who is starting to feel hungry. When my teens have to wait more than about 30 minutes past their normal dinner time, they become anxious and aggressive. Remember, babies are just smaller versions of us with much smaller stomachs than my teenagers.

Sometimes hunger is not triggered by physical pain but rather other stimuli. As feeding time nears, the **smell of the mother** and her breastmilk can trigger hunger – much like your appetite may be piqued if you walk into a house where a pie is baking or bacon is frying.

Babies may also want to suck if they are **anxious, scared** or even occasionally **bored** – similar to our own **comfort eating**. You can introduce a pacifier (dummy) to help calm a baby that is not hungry but wants oral (sucking) comfort; however it is *suggested* that you wait until the four week mark in order to avoid confusion, frustration or preference. Babies need to learn how to feed well at the breast before you introduce anything else into their mouths.

MONITOR BREAST FULLNESS

Often it is the mother's own body that tells her that it is feeding time. It is not uncommon for the mother to wake up with slightly **engorged** or **leaking** breasts that tell her the baby will need to feed soon. Even if a baby is still asleep, it may be time to start arousing them to feed by holding them skin to skin. Taking some milk out to avoid pain (with a hand pump or using hand expression) can help if the baby is expected to wake shortly.

It is fascinating to see the mother's body working in harmony with the baby's feeding routine. Many women report waking in the night just seconds before their baby starts to wake – as if a silent alarm clock has gone off for both the mother and baby.

OFFER APPETIZER, ENTRÉE AND DESSERT!

Remember that not all milk coming out of the breast is created equal. In the first few minutes, the baby is receiving the higher lactose, lower fat and less caloric **foremilk** that is needed for brain development and to quench his thirst. I refer to the foremilk as the ***appetizer***. After several minutes, the baby starts to receive the higher fat hindmilk ***from the same breast*** which is vital for growth and helping the baby feel satisfied. I refer to the hindmilk as the **entreé**.

It is important that the baby feeds long enough on the breast to receive both foremilk and hindmilk. A baby who is swapped to the 2nd breast after a few minutes is not getting to the hindmilk and not emptying the mother's breast. The other issue with moving a baby from one breast to the other after only a few minutes is that the baby is only receiving foremilk and will want to feed a lot more often – never feeling fully satisfied. These babies may also end up losing some weight as they are not taking in the fatty milk that is needed for weight gain.

In addition, a baby who receives mostly foremilk may find their stomach easily irritated. Excessive foremilk can cause him to spit up a lot, have frothy explosive green diapers, experience pain and crying from a gassy stomach and/or have slower weight gain. Aim to **hit the hindmilk** by keeping the baby on the first breast as long as possible (at least 10 minutes). In the early days of breastfeeding, babies may feed for much longer on the first breast.

I refer to the 2nd breast during the same feed as ***dessert***. Just like in a restaurant, you may feel full after you have eaten the appetizer and entree but if you wait a while, you might find room for dessert. Always offer the baby the 2nd breast (*dessert*) after 5-10 minutes. If the baby doesn't want any more, that is OK. At the next feed, start with the breast that would have been ***dessert*** on the last feed.

Women have come up with crafty ways to remember which breast to start on at the next feed. Many mothers will move a bracelet or ring on to the left or right arm or hand in order to remind her which breast to start on next time. Some use a bow or clip on the *dessert* bra strap. And of course there are now plenty of apps to help you remember. That breast will probably feel fuller at the next feed as well. Partners also seem to have a weird knack for remembering which side you fed from last.

LOOK FOR SIGNS OF BEING FULL

When adults start to feel full, the first noticeable sign is usually a *slowdown in chewing and swallowing*. Babies are similar – they tend to suck quickly at first in order to trigger let down and then slow down their suck pattern as they transfer milk from the breast to their stomach. When they feel full, they *stop sucking and often unlatch independently*. I jokingly say that a full breastfed newborn looks like 'drunk uncle during the holidays' – a glassy eyed look along with somewhat of a vacant stare and the desire to *doze off*.

An older baby will not fall asleep immediately after a feed but will have relaxed (unclenched) hands and feet. Assuming the baby is not in pain from an air pocket or gas bubble, the full baby will probably be calm, alert and even playful until his next nap time.

Remember that what goes in must also come out and a baby that is having a *consistent number of wet and dirty diapers* in the early days is clearly getting enough. Newborn babies often fill a diaper right after a feed. *As the baby grows, it is not uncommon for an older baby (8+ weeks) to go for a day (or several) without dirtying his or her diaper*. Of course the real evidence of a baby getting enough is that they are *gaining adequate weight*.

Finally, a mother can often tell that her baby has had enough because her breasts 'feel empty'. While this is not a foolproof sign – as many mothers who feel this way can hand express another ounce or have a baby who wants to feed more ten minutes later – it is an instinctive gauge.

DIAPER COUNTS

HOW MANY?	Day 1	Day 2	Day 3	Day 4	Day 5	Day 6	Day 7
*Expected Wet Diapers	1	2	3	5+	6+	6+	6+
*Expected Dirty Diapers	1	2	3	3+	3+	3+	3+

*These are guidelines. Some babies have more or less than the quoted minimum. However a baby who is not getting enough milk often has far fewer diapers.

MEET THE GAS BROTHERS: BURP, RUMBLE & FART

Getting used to a baby's bodily cues can take time but most parents recognize the sound of a burp, rumbling tummy or a fart. Burps are bursts of swallowed air that come back up from the stomach and out of the mouth as a mixture of oxygen and nitrogen ('gas'). Some babies swallow more air than others; breastfed babies swallow very little air when feeding compared to bottle fed ones. All babies take in air when crying. After feeding on one breast, most mothers will burp a baby to ward off pain, make room for a little more milk and help avoid spitting some back. If your baby spits up a bit of milk after a feed, it is likely that this was caused by an escaping bubble that pushed some milk out of a very full baby.

In order to burp the infant, sit your baby on your lap and support their body and head by aligning your thumb and forefinger with the baby's lower jawbone in a V (see next page). This can feel awkward but gives good support and frees up the other hand to pat or rub the baby's back (around the bottom of his/her ribcage) in order to attempt to release gas. The burp hold should not touch the baby's neck or throat.

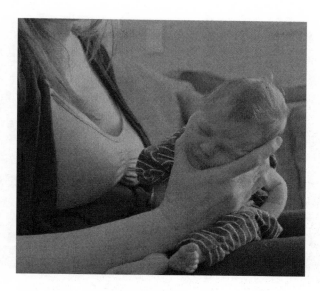

The V Hold for Burping

A rumbly tummy is often the sign of gas on its way to passing through the other end of the baby and is referred to as flatulence or farting. Babies are usually skilled at doing this on their own but movement (light downward tummy massage or a slow bicycling of the legs) can assist. Many babies find lower gas painful until it is released. Usually a baby clears gas by itself but some are better at doing so than others.

There are a few products on the market aimed at relieving gas either by breaking down the bubbles into a smaller size (simethicone drops), helping the anal sphincter open up (the Windi®) or soothe the discomfort (gripe water). All three have benefits and risks which should be weighed. Gripe water is controversial and results are mixed. All regulatory bodies believe that no liquid - other than breastmilk or formula - should be introduced into babies less than six months of age.

WAKE A SLEEPY (DEHYDRATED?) BABY

Some babies do not wake when their stomachs are empty – their bodily signal has not quite adjusted to life on the outside yet. Anyone who tells you that their *newborn* slept for six hours at a time probably did not realize that they had a baby who was possibly severely dehydrated and in danger of decline. You do not need to wake a baby that is stable and gaining roughly an ounce a day (5-7 oz. per week). However, babies born below the 15 percentile for weight or weighing less than five pounds (approx. 2500g) will probably need to be woken to feed. The same goes for babies who are not gaining weight and/or have jaundice on Day 3. These babies may be in danger if we do not wake them to feed.

It can be especially difficult to wake a sleepy baby. Try taking off blankets or clothing to let cool air awaken them. The mother's body temperature adjusts to regulate the baby's temperature when they are skin to skin. Changing their diaper (or at least letting air circulate under a diaper) can also wake them up a bit. Rubbing (or in the case of my pediatrician friend 'flicking') the bottom of the baby's foot can arouse him. Finally, using different feeding positions or plopping a drop of breast milk on the baby's lip can often wake up the baby.

If the baby falls asleep after a few minutes of feeding, you can try burping them to arouse them. Another tip for provoking a baby to take a little more milk from the breast is to gently lift the baby's arm (at the wrist) into a full stretch and then gently bringing the arm back down into resting position (pg. 100). This raising of the arm often causes bursts of sucking – sort of like pulling the arm of a pinball machine fires the ball.

SUMMARY

☐ Cues (signs) that a baby is hungry include lip, tongue and mouth movement, movement of the hands and feet, and rooting for the breast. Crying is a late sign that the baby is very hungry.

☐ Breast fullness or engorgement is usually a sign that the baby needs to feed. Removing a little milk by hand expressing or pumping can help with engorgement and an easier latch.

☐ Feed the baby on the first breast for 10-25 minutes in order to break through into the more satisfying hindmilk and empty the breast as much as possible. Always offer the 2nd breast (*dessert*) at the feed. Start the next feed on the breast that would have been *dessert* on the last feed.

☐ A baby that receives too much foremilk may exhibit symptoms of colic (see pg. 144).

☐ Signs that a baby is full or had enough to eat include adequate weight gain, a consistent number of wet and dirty diapers, a baby slowing down their sucking and swallowing, unclenched hands, unlatching independently and/or dozing off. Older babies become calm after a feed and often benefit from some playtime.

☐ Air trapped in a baby's stomach or intestines is usually burped back through the mouth or farted out through the anal sphincter. Burping is done to coax an air bubble out, relieve pain or make room for a little more milk. Breastfed babies do not take in as much air as bottle fed babies and may not burp as much in the first few weeks.

☐ Babies that are jaundiced or not gaining weight should be woken for feeds in the day and night if they are not waking naturally. Taking off some clothes, putting a drop or two of breastmilk on the baby's lip or rubbing the baby's feet may help wake up the baby.

LATOYA'S STORY – READ THE SIGNS

I was the youngest child in my family and I never remember seeing a woman breastfeed except in a book my mom had. Deciding to 'nurse' (as my stepmom called it) seemed the right thing to do and I remember Salisha self-attaching to me right after birth. It felt weird – like a fish was nibbling on me at first.

We got off to a good start but I had a sleepy baby on my hands and it never occurred to me to wake her up. I just figured that she'd wake up and cry when she was hungry. On the 2nd night, she slept for six hours straight and I thought she was going to be an easy baby. She seemed to be on the breast for a very long time when she was feeding so I didn't worry about it – well until the doctor weighed her at one week and told me that she wasn't gaining weight fast enough.

He asked me lots of questions about her eating and sleeping habits and it was only when he told me that I should be feeding her 8-10 times a day that I realized why she was losing weight. She would turn her head toward the breast and root. She would get fidgety and move her feet. She'd stick her tongue out a lot. Now I know that those were signs of hunger. But then, I just thought they were cute baby behaviors and waited until she cried to feed her.

I also fed her from both breasts switching every couple minutes. My milk supply decreased and the baby had some nasty green diapers. After talking to the lactation consultant, I know to empty one breast completely and it's OK if she doesn't want the second. Things are calming down for us now and breastfeeding is getting easier. My advice to you mammas is to know the signs and don't stop learning about breastfeeding!

AUTHOR'S NOTE: If you haven't been raised around babies, the first several months are full of learning curves. Latoya now has three children and has never stopped learning.

CHAPTER 6

ATTACH & LATCH A BABY TO THE BREAST (PARTNER*)

***BREASTFEEDING DOESN'T HAVE TO SUCK** if the baby is well positioned, following 'The Rules' and latches on deeply at the right angle.*

Women who have mastered breastfeeding make it look easy. They often multitask with a baby feeding on one breast while they are talking on the phone, stirring a sauce or dealing with a toddler on the potty. But in the beginning, just like driving a car, breastfeeding can be daunting and may require help to overcome problems. This chapter highlights the basic rules of breastfeeding, the mechanics of a deep latch and techniques you can try if latching is causing you pain. A good latch should not hurt.

FOLLOW TWO RULES

The first rule of breastfeeding is to put the baby *tummy to tummy (or front to front)* with the mother in most every position. This may seem very obvious but when you are handed a newborn and have never breastfed before, you may naturally cradle the baby in your arm so the baby is looking up at you and assume the baby will turn her head into the breast. While a baby can feed with her head turned at a 90° angle, it is much harder to eat this way. I compare it to putting a sandwich by your ear and then asking you to take a bite. It is much easier if the sandwich is in front of your nose and mouth. You can then see it, smell it, open wide and lean forward to take a bite.

Once you are tummy to tummy with your baby, **the 2nd *rule*** of breastfeeding is to start by putting your nipple just below the baby's nose (***nose to nipple***). This rule always seemed odd to me until I realized that nose to nipple forces the baby to reach up with his jaw and mouth open wide. The latch is far more effective if the baby pushes his **chin slightly outward** to attach to the breast. By starting the baby nose to nipple, you are encouraging that chin out, head up attachment.

Remember that babies cannot open wide if you are pushing or controlling their head or neck towards the breast; they need to be able to rock their head back slightly and lunge forward. Support his or her body with your hand across his neck, back and shoulders if the baby is lying horizontally. If the baby is vertical or diagonal across the mother, support the baby's head with fingers behind the baby's ears.

A GOOD LATCH IS LIKE A SHARK ENCOUNTER

Latch is the word used to describe how the baby attaches to the breast to remove milk. My partner used to compare the baby latching on to the breast to a *shark attacking its prey*. Like babies, sharks sense their food is nearby through smell. Once they have located approximately where that food is, the shark shuts his eyes, opens his mouth wide and reaches up to scoop in as much food as possible. When a baby senses the nipple is within reach, she also opens her mouth wide in anticipation.

Remember to bring the baby to the breast **chin first** so that the nipple is angled slightly upward (at about 45°) towards the roof of the baby's mouth. When the baby opens his or her mouth to its widest point, latch the baby quickly.

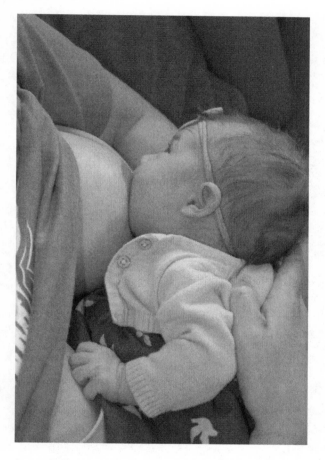

A great latch: chin first, slight tilt of the head back and the bottom of the areola covered more than the top. ©M.A. Cockeram

You are not trying to get the entire areola into the baby's mouth. Instead, aim for the baby to latch on to the nipple and areola covering **more of the bottom of the areola than the top**. The baby's upper and lower lip should flare out slightly to create a good seal.

The angle of the nipple in the baby's mouth is crucial for preventing nipple damage. If the nipple goes into the baby' mouth pointing slightly upward (*'nipple north'*), it has a better chance of being pulled up and stretched back against the soft palate (which is made of muscle). Damage is caused when the nipple gets trapped between the baby's tongue (which moves back and forth) and the hard palate (which is made of bone). Feel the difference between the boney hard palate and the muscular soft palate by taking your tongue behind your front teeth, moving up into the roof of your mouth and throat and then suddenly reaching the silky soft palate (aka the comfort zone). ***Remember, a deep latch rarely hurts***.

If you feel that the latch is shallow, use your little finger to break the baby's suction and try again. During the first 30 seconds of the latch, you can assist let down by **massaging around the top of the breast** (about 1-2 inches from the baby's face once latched). Like teenagers, babies want instant gratification and waiting for the milk to flow can be frustrating. A little massage of gentle circles with your knuckle can get let down going a little bit faster. Some women let down very quickly – leading to the baby coughing or splattering as milk sprays into their mouth at speed.

A baby with a weak suck, restricted tongue movement, the inability to flare out his lips or who latches at a nose first (instead of chin first) angle is a baby that will probably cause his mother soreness or damage. Not all babies can manage to get the breast deep enough in his or her mouth to allow pain-free breastfeeding *initially*. But usually with a few adjustments to position and latch, babies can feed more efficiently and cause little or no pain to their mothers.

AVOID THE NIPPLE TRAP - SANDWICH AND FLIPPLE!

As mentioned previously, the nipple *stretches* as it is stimulated by sucking. A nipple that gets trapped between the hard palate and the tongue is easily damaged. While bringing the baby to the breast chin first often alleviates a shallow latch, many mothers take positioning a step further.

The 'Sandwich and Flipple' technique helps many women to avoid the *nipple trap* by helping to angle the nipple upwards into a small mouth. First, *sandwich* the areola by gathering a tiny bit of skin and areola in your hand. This flattened (sandwiched) skin is easier for the baby to latch on to compared to a wider area.

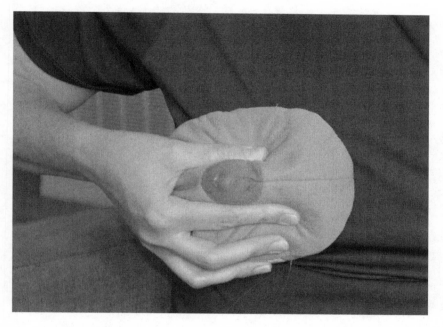

Sandwiching for upright feeding positions (laid back, supine, side-lying, etc.) ©M Cockeram 2019

Next, gently push down on the sandwiched skin right above the areola with your thumb and **FLIPPLE (flip the nipple)** upwards a bit towards your own chin. As the baby opens wide to latch, you let go of the skin and flip the nipple up and forward, assisting it into the top and back of the baby's mouth. If you can master it – and it takes a little practice – you will achieve a deeper and wider latch.

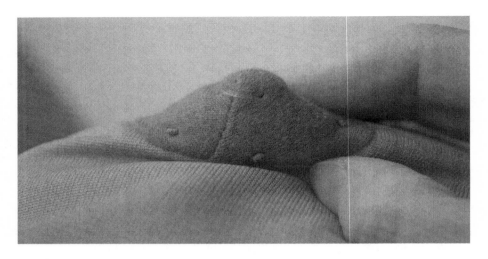

Sandwich followed by the flipple. ©M Cockeram 2019

TRICK: Think of how you would push down on a burger to make it easier to take a bite. This is the same principle for **sandwiching** the nipple in order for the baby to latch easier.

If the baby is lying horizontally across your body, you will need to squeeze the breast vertically (from the sides) and flipple away from the baby's mouth before releasing.

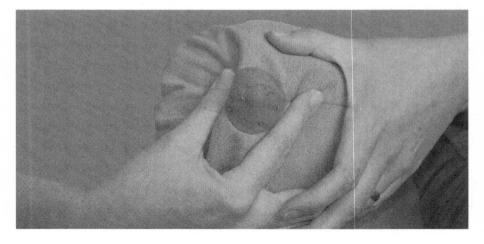

Sandwiching for horizontal feeding positions (cradle, cross cradle, football, etc.). ©M Cockeram 2019

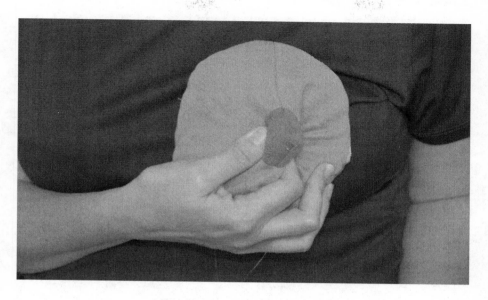

...followed by the flipple. ©M Cockeram 2019

Think of the flipple like putting the breast into the baby's mouth **starting from the bottom of the areola and then letting the rest of the breast roll forward** with the nipple flipping into the baby's mouth last. Your goal is to get as much of the nipple and areola high and deep into the baby's mouth so that the tongue rubs the bottom of the areola instead of the bottom of nipple and avoids damage.

IS IT ENGORGEMENT OR WATER RETENTION?

As mentioned in Chapter 3, many women suffer from swelling in the first few days as a result of the water they are retaining from the fluids they received in labor. This fluid lands in anything that hangs down (ankles, wrists, breasts, etc.) and is referred to as *third spacing*. A breast retaining water can be mistaken for an **engorged** one. Engorged breasts are warm, feel the firmness of your arm and don't alter the nipple while breasts **swollen from fluid retention tend to pull the nipple inward and feel more like a water balloon to the**

touch. In order to help a baby latch on to a breast retaining water, a technique called **reverse pressure softening** is used to evert the nipple and areola. It is similar to making a (smaller) sandwich with the breast but encourages the nipple to protrude out of the areola.

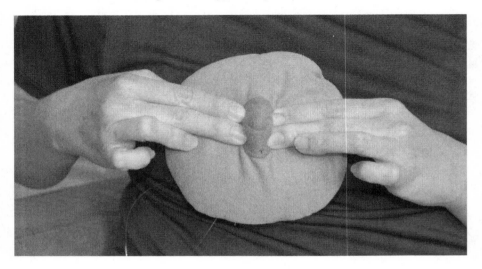

Reverse Pressure Softening ©M Cockeram 2019

USE A NIPPLE SHIELD OR EVERTER

Nipple soreness is almost always the result of a baby's shallow latch. While we can try many things in order to correct the problem, injured, bleeding nipples are enough to make any woman want to quit breastfeeding. One of the short term workarounds is a **nipple shield**. In addition to a shallow latch, babies born prematurely or sleepy eaters may benefit from a nipple shield because it helps the baby learn to use his/her tongue to draw the nipple into the mouth. It also allows for a better grip. Women who have flat or inverted nipples may also find nipple shields very helpful.

Just like most bodily items, nipple shields come in *different sizes (16mm, 20mm & 24mm)* so it is essential that it fits the mother's breast and allows the baby to draw the nipple up. A lactation consultant can easily recommend the right size for you. By turning the edge of the shield inside out, it is easy to place over the nipple for the deepest fit. Then flip the edges back to affix. Many women use lanolin cream or breast milk drops along the edge of the shield to create a better seal.

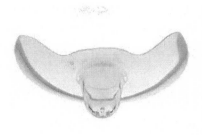

Nipple Shield

Inverted (non-protruding) nipples may (or may not) present a problem depending upon the severity (Grade 1-3) of the inversion. Some inverted nipples pop out easily when a baby latches on to the breast, others don't.

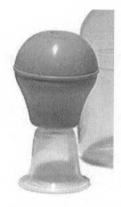

You can make a nipple prominent using an Everter (pictured). This simple suction device is first squeezed, then placed on top of the areola and then released. The suction usually draws the nipple out easily. If your nipple is inverted, do not worry about breastfeeding right now. A lactation educator or consultant can help you once the baby is here and you may not have a problem.

BE ON THE LOOKOUT FOR A TONGUE (OR LIP) TIE

Many mothers will have a baby that causes nipple pain when feeding because the baby has a short or tight *lingual frenulum*. The frenulum is the band of tissue that attaches the bottom of the tongue to the bottom of the mouth. A tongue needs a good degree of movement both upward and side to side in order to latch to the breast. A frenulum that is short, thick or tight –*referred to as a **tongue tie or ankyloglossia*** - restricts the baby's tongue movement and can cause a shallow latch. An anterior tongue tie means that the frenulum attaches

79

to the tongue closer to the tip. A posterior tie means that the frenulum attaches at the base of the tongue. In some severe cases, a tongue tie can impair speech.

Symptoms of a tongue tie include a clicking noise when feeding, gas or reflux, the baby 'sliding' off the breast or trouble keeping grasp of the breast, the baby unlatching quickly and crying in frustration or getting tired quickly when breastfeeding or a quivering jaw after a feed. Mothers may notice that their nipple looks lipstick shaped – often with a white stripe from being pinched or experience a vasospasm (pg. 139-140) and experience plugged ducts or mastitis more frequently.

If you suspect a problem, see a lactation consultant early for a referral. A procedure called a frenotomy (aka revision or frenuloplasty) can be performed that lengthens the frenulum and allows for more tongue movement. The procedure is normally performed within the first 30 days of birth.

The upper lip also has a frenulum (*labial frenulum*) that can present problems when breastfeeding if it is tight (***lip tie***) because babies flare out their upper and lower lips in order to make a good seal on the breast. While a similar procedure can be performed on the lip tie, ***it is far more controversial*** as to the difference it could make on the depth of the latch. Again, talk to your child's care provider early to see if a lip tie procedure is a consideration. Sometimes severe lip ties result in a gap between the child's two front teeth.

If the baby has a lip or tongue tie correction, their gum or mouth may be sore for the first few days and this could lead to a ***breastfeeding strike*** since the baby associates feeding with pain. If the baby is pulling off the breast in pain, consider pumping for a day or two until healing begins and spend as much time skin to skin as possible.

SUMMARY:

☐ Put the baby **tummy to tummy** and **baby's nose close to mom's nipple** as you get ready to feed. The baby should scoop the breast in from below, lifting her chin up as she latches. Never push or support the baby onto the breast with the crown of his or her head. The baby needs to be able to move his or her head to open the mouth wide.

☐ **Massaging the breast** before or during feeding can stimulate the milk ejection reflex (aka *let down*).

☐ A **deep latch** is when the baby is able to stretch the nipple down the throat to the **muscular** soft palate and usually does not cause the mother any pain.

☐ A **shallow latch** results from the baby not being able to pull the stretchy nipple past the **boney** hard palate. This is often caused by poor positioning, the shape or strength of the baby's mouth, tongue or lips. If it hurts, try re-latching.

☐ *Sandwiching* the breast can make it easier for a baby to latch. If engorged, removing some milk by hand expressing can soften a hard breast and allow an easier latch.

☐ *The flipple* is a technique where you unroll the breast into the baby's mouth starting with the bottom of the areola and flipping the nipple into the baby's mouth last. This technique can secure a deeper and wider latch.

☐ If the breast is swollen from fluid retention, the reverse pressure softening technique can ease latching.

☐ Using a nipple shield can be an excellent <u>short term</u> solution if damage occurs from a shallow latch. Shields come in different sizes.

☐A nipple everter can help an inverted nipple become prominent so the baby can latch easier.

☐Tongue (and possibly lip ties) can cause a painful latch. A procedure can be done to lengthen the tongue's frenulum which allows better freedom of movement and a deeper latch. Watch for symptoms and talk to your care provider early if you feel the baby may have this impairment.

EZRA'S TONGUE TIE STORY

In April, I had my fourth baby – a sweet boy we named Ezra. I was convinced breastfeeding would be a cinch because I had already done it for 11 years with my other children. Fast forward to 10pm at night on Day three: Ezra was screaming on my lap as I watched How-To-Latch videos through tearful eyes. Both of my extra-pink nipples bore a horizontal stripe of raw, rubbed openness coupled with tiny scabs. With every suck, I tightened and cringed and cried with pain. I labeled him a bad nurser. I tried dragging the nipple down his face and over his nose, using the teacup hold of the nipple, the "flipple", and even the laid-back breastfeeding position. I tried a nipple shield that, incidentally, made it worse. Nothing worked.

After a few weeks, I was still in great pain but the physical damage to my nipples was not getting worse, and that gave me hope. I found some Hydrogel Pads I had gotten as samples once and they helped with the healing. I figured out by latching him in football hold, nursing sessions became bearable. We also nursed lying down at night using a small light to latch and re-latch when it got too painful (and it was never not painful). I continued looking for answers.

Besides the pain of breastfeeding, Ezra gained weight like crazy - 38 ounces in 21 days. He did spit up A LOT – milk flying out of his mouth in arching streams. Keeping the nipple in his mouth was difficult, as it would constantly slide out unless I held my breast in place. Once in a while when the nipple neared his lips, this disgusted look would appear on his face, as if I had presented him with something rotten and he would slowly chew his way up the nipple to latch. And as he nursed, he clicked like a horse trotting on pavement.

Armed with a digital camera, I took pictures of this baby every day. When he was 3 weeks old I was scrolling through the latest batch, and suddenly, there it was: Ezra was crying, eyes shut, mouth open, with a tongue that **curled and cupped up**. I recognized that to be a posterior tongue-tie (PTT)! Although I had worked with breastfeeding moms for ten years, I had not experienced a baby with one. Once I saw that picture, I posted it on Facebook and sent it to a lactation specialist friend and thought to myself "Maybe he's not a bad nurser after all!?"

When we speak of tongue-ties, we normally mean anterior tongue-ties, the obvious tethered (often heart-shaped) tongue - easy to spot - that could be clipped in a simple office procedure. My lactation consultant friend used the term "stingray tongue" to describe Ezra's PTT. By the time we met with the specialist doctor three weeks later, I was certain Ezra had an upper lip-tie, posterior tongue-tie and high-arch palate. All three of my suspicions were confirmed. This doctor agreed to fix the PTT but was not a believer in touching upper lip-ties. By using scissors, a diamond-shaped cut under the tongue would give it more mobility and hopefully make breastfeeding better for us. I left satisfied with the diagnosis and proposed treatment.

While waiting out the next appointment, I found a fabulous resource of understanding: the Tongue Tie Babies Support Group on Facebook. There I learned that many professionals do not know how to identify ties (especially PTTs) nor do many believe in correcting ties - especially in infants. Few professionals believe that ties can interfere with feeding, speech or digestion either. I have seen that many different kinds of professionals treat ties, from pediatricians to dentists to ENTs and GPs -- there isn't one kind of doctor who specializes in this area. While some doctors fix ties with scissors, others prefer to use lasers. Some breastfeeding moms notice immediate relief and change; others report it takes weeks for things to feel better.

Doing more research, I decided to get a 2nd opinion. I wasn't convinced that using scissors was the way to go. I also wasn't sure that the upper lip tie didn't play a bigger role in the problem. The Doctor that I chose for this was a dentist that uses laser treatment. The Dentist examined Ezra and agreed that we could benefit from having the ties revised. He explained the procedure and we got under way immediately. After numbing Ezra's mouth, the procedure took less than five minutes. Ezra cried and moved a lot, but I knew he was probably more bothered by the restraining of his head than the laser surgery. There was a little blood but that was it!

I tried to latch him after ten minutes of recovery but Ezra's numb mouth made latching difficult. At lunch I nursed Ezra for the first time. I could already see a part of his upper lip turned out that I had never seen before – it wasn't a huge flanging or anything, but it was something. I did not notice relief though – if anything it felt a little worse. Thirty minutes later, Ezra had a small meltdown. He would try to latch but I could tell he was in pain. I had been told that he might not want to nurse too much in the first 24 hours, so it wasn't a surprise. I gave him Tylenol and an hour later he settled down to nurse. I still couldn't tell a difference in my pain level.

I gave him one more dose of Tylenol later that evening and, by the next afternoon, he seemed back to normal. The doctor had instructed us to stretch the upper lip and sweep under the tongue once every hour Ezra was awake. Ezra's "reflux" stopped almost overnight. He would still spit up, but it was nothing like before. His clicking was mostly gone. That strange (cute) way he had of chewing up to latch on the nipple with a grimace on his face was gone, as was his way of sliding off the nipple while nursing.

Sadly I wasn't noticing much change. Although some women note instant relief after their babies' revisions, it seemed to me that for everyone who had that experience, there were four women who said it took many weeks for full effect so I kept up with the exercises and encouraged wider and deeper latching. Two weeks passed and I wasn't feeling better. The nipple shape still showed some compression stripes after nursing. I tried to be patient, continued with the stretches, and kept correcting shallow latches. Around three weeks, I started to feel a shift. By four weeks, I could safely say I believed we were cured. It was a long journey but we got there in the end.

AUTHOR'S NOTE: The story of the diagnosis and treatment of Ezra's posterior tongue tie was quite a learning curve. If you are experiencing pain and nipple damage, a 'clicking' noise when the baby breastfeeds or the baby sliding off the nipple or struggling to latch, have a look at his or her tongue. If you suspect the baby may have a tongue or lip tie, get (well-researched) help as soon as possible.

CHAPTER 7

GET INTO POSITION TO FEED COMFORTABLY

BREASTFEEDING DOESN'T HAVE TO SUCK *if you can find breastfeeding positions that work for both of you.*

Like labor, being in a good comfortable position makes everything easier for both the mother and baby. The important thing is to be in a position in which you feel confident and that doesn't strain any part of you. Don't let anyone tell you what position is *best* for you. Use the ones that work for you. It is also useful to have a **large *glass of water* (with straw) within reach** when breastfeeding. Many women feel a sudden thirst when they let down.

GET IN POSITION

In the hospital during the golden hour(s) after the birth (and if recovering from a C-section), many women will be encouraged to latch the baby to breast with the baby lying on top of the mother. This is referred to as **biological nursing** (also called **frontal, supine, semi-reclining or laid-back feeding)** and is probably the most natural mammalian feeding position of all. It allows the baby to self-attach using the pendulum-like swinging and bobbing of the head and requires little support from the mother. This positioning allows the curves of the baby and mother to happily mold together as a unit.

The big advantage of having the baby lying on the mother is that the baby is on top of the food source and gravity can help a small mouth fill up with as much breast as possible. Gravity also helps the baby maintain his or her position without the help of the mother's arms or hands. If a baby is ever refusing the breast, this position may solve the problem. This position gives the baby complete control from the start. Use this position for as long as you both feel comfortable.

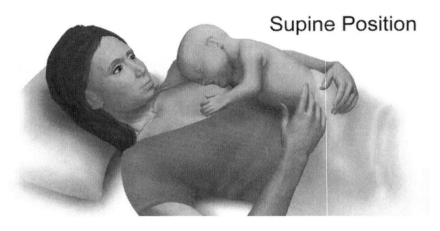

Supine Position

Courtesy of BruceBlaus

When the mother comes home from the hospital, she is much more likely to be feeding in a *sitting position* since we tend to stay out of the bedroom during the daytime. Most sitting positions encourage the mother to have her back straight, feet slightly elevated on a small stool and often using pillows or cushions to raise the baby's body close to the breasts.

The most common new mom sitting position is called the **Cross Cradle**. In this position you sit comfortably with a straight back, feet flat or elevated slightly on a stool and with the baby lying across you diagonally or parallel with the breasts. Then you use both hands: one hand supports and controls the breast and the other hand supports the baby. The baby should be tummy to tummy rather than having to turn his or her head. Be careful not to limit the baby's head as he needs freedom of movement to latch.

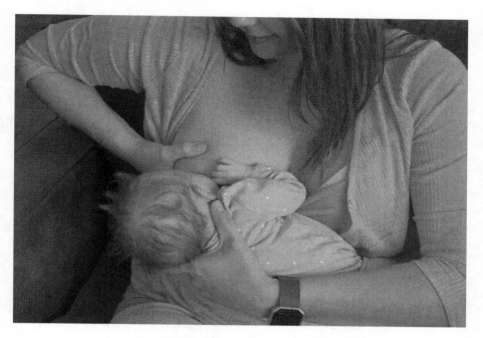

The Cross Cradle. ©M Cockeram 2019

> **TIP:** The Cross Cradle is often easier when you use a breastfeeding pillow or cushion under the baby's body. You can also wear a cover up if breastfeeding in front of others is intimidating.

A variation of the cross cradle is called the **cradle position**. It is a one handed hold (pg. 90) and is usually used with slightly older babies who have established neck control. The bend in your arm cradles the baby's head.

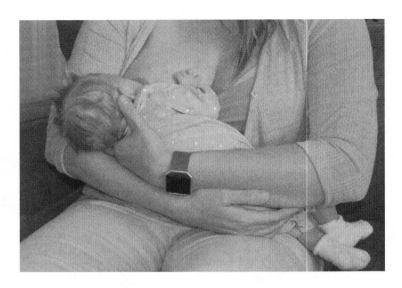

The Cradle. ©M Cockeram 2019

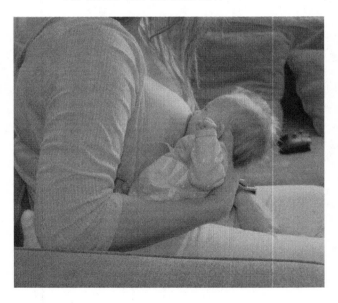

The Football Hold. ©M Cockeram 2019

Another popular position is called the **Football (or Rugby ball) hold** named for the way a player carries the ball. Many women (and lactation consultants) favor this one-handed position because they find it easier to latch the baby and they can see his expression, eyes, latch, etc. It can also be useful for feeding twins at the same time. Be careful not to limit the baby's head or neck movement in this position. It can feel awkward at first and can take practice to get it right for both of you.

The Semi-reclining position is an instinctive mammalian feeding position. With the baby sitting and facing you (bolstered up by cushions if not high enough to reach the breast), the baby latches on the same way you'd eat a sandwich: with the food out in front of you. Many babies feed this way while being carried in a sling and usually need very little help.

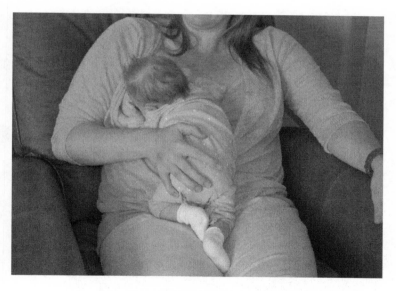

Semi-Reclining. ©M Cockeram 2019

FEED FLAT AT NIGHT

Several feeds at night (between 10pm-6am) are usually necessary in the first several weeks and months of having a newborn. The mother's milk supply rejuvenates when she is sleeping and is usually plentiful overnight. The baby often feeds quickly and goes back to sleep easier if not fully woken by bright lights or cold air. It is easy however to form a bad latch when it is dark and you are tired. A small bedside flashlight can be handy for checking the latch without fully waking up the baby. Mobile phones flashlight apps are also useful but tend to be far brighter than needed.

Some women feel they should take the baby out of the bedroom when feeding at night so no one else is woken or disturbed. Moving to a soft comfy chair or sofa can be tempting but it can also be a danger zone for a baby whose mother falls asleep. If the mother dozes off, the baby could slide down into a cramped space and may not be able to dislocate himself without help. The best place to feed the baby when you are tired is on a flat surface and a bed is the natural solution at night.

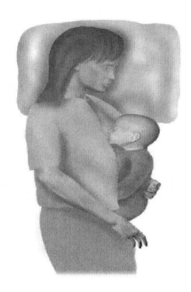

Side-Lying Position

Courtesy of Bruce Blaus

The **side-lying position (aka the dream feeding position**) is the most commonly used night time feeding position. You may also find that one breast is usually enough during the night. Curled up and warm together, it is easy for both of you to fall back asleep.

Although breastfed babies are significantly less likely to be affected by Sudden Infant Death Syndrome (SIDS), the American Association of Pediatrics (AAP, 2011) recommends putting the baby *back to sleep* on his back on a firm surface, having the baby **sleep** in the same room (but not in the same bed) and keeping excess blankets, pillows, etc. away from the baby's body. Using a bedside bassinet, a co-sleeper that attaches to the mother's side of the bed or a separate crib are thought to be the safest solutions.

For many reasons, mothers are not always willing or able to put their baby in a separate space after feeding. Some babies will not settle without knowing their mother is next to them. It is not uncommon for babies to sleep on a mother or partner's chest in the first few days or weeks after birth. In fact, bed sharing/co-sleeping is common practice in most all countries of the world and is probably more common in the USA then documented because of the stigma associated with not following the AAP recommendation. If you want to sleep together in the safest possible way, consider the following:

- Avoid bed sharing/co-sleeping with a <u>formula</u> fed baby.
- Avoid bed sharing/co-sleeping with a baby less than 5lbs or born prematurely.
- Avoid bed sharing/co-sleeping if the mother is morbidly **obese**, has been **drinking alcohol, smoking or taking drugs** which would weaken or impair her instincts.

Assuming none of the aforementioned conditions apply, the safest way to bed-share is to keep the baby on the mother's side (i.e. not in the middle of the bed between two adults) *until at least six months* of age. Studies of co-sleeping mothers and babies show that women who are sober and breastfeeding at night tend to sleep facing each other at about breast level. Interestingly, the mother often creates a *protective C* shape around their baby with one arm.

Partners do not necessarily have the same instinct – especially if they are not sober. So if you are sleeping with your baby between the two of you and your partner is under the influence of anything that could alter his or her primal instincts, consider co-sleeping with the baby in another room or ask the partner to relocate.

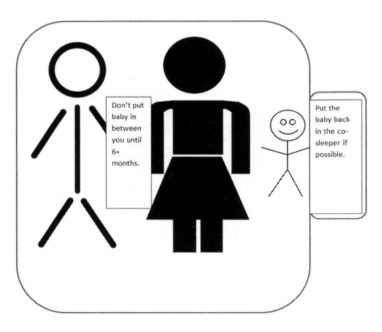

Safe Sleeping Arrangements

SUMMARY:

☐ In the early days of breastfeeding, having a baby lying directly on top of the breast (frontal/semi-reclining) may be easier for both of you. It is the most instinctive mammalian feeding position.

☐ There are many other breastfeeding positions including cross cradle, semi-reclining, side-lying and football. Try different positions and use the one that feels comfortable and results in an effective latch.

☐ The cross cradle position is the most common one for new mothers. The fingers of one hand guide the baby's neck; the other hand supports the breast.

☐ Although you may feel you need to take the baby to a separate room to feed him/her at night, beware of falling asleep on stuffed furniture where the baby could slide down and get stuck between cushions, etc.

☐ While co-sleeping/bed-sharing is not recommended by the AAP due to increased SIDS risk, there are ways to make sleeping together safer including using a bassinet next to the bed or keeping the baby on the mother's side of the bed until six months of age.

BLAKES STORY – I NEVER INTENDED TO CO-SLEEP!

I had not intended to have a baby in the bed with us. I had a great deal of fear instilled in me from news stories, family members, and friends about the potential dangers of sleeping together. We got the baby room ready with a crib – fully intending that Jack would sleep there at night on his own after the first few months.

Unfortunately Jack was a very colicky baby and was awake every two hours at night for several weeks. I became exhausted very quickly after the birth and realized that I was falling asleep on the sofa when he latched during night feeds. One night he actually pushed off of me and fell on the floor. He was not injured but it really scared me and made me realize that something needed to change.

That was the point at which I decided I'd better do my research about co-sleeping and feeding in bed. Feeding on a flat surface seemed far safer than on a sofa or chair in the middle of the night. I learned that Sudden Infant Death Syndrome (SIDS) is significantly reduced in exclusively breastfed babies and two-thirds of the world's babies co-sleep with their mothers every night. I also read that there are definitely ways to make co-sleeping safer. My care providers (for both children) were actually laid back when I told them that I was bed sharing. We kept an open dialogue about it during visits.

First of all I started wearing a sweatshirt to bed so I wouldn't need a comforter or blanket over both of us. I always kept Jack on my side of the bed – not in between my husband and me - until he was much older. I know it may sound impossible but I was (and still am) completely aware of him in bed at all times. All he wanted was to be next to me to absorb my warmth and smell (and milk if hungry).

There came a point in which he was 'sleeping through' and did not need to feed in the night anymore. We tried putting him down to sleep in his crib but he wanted no part of it. I just couldn't let him cry either – it tore me up. Eventually around the nine month mark I just embraced bed sharing permanently. Once I did embrace my decision, it was so much easier. This may not be the right decision for everybody but it was definitely what worked best for me and my family. I think there is a lot of fear about bed sharing that is unfounded. Current research is pointing to neurological issues being the potential cause of SIDS, not co-sleeping. Time will tell.

I called Jack my 'trial and error baby'. When Henry came along four years later, I didn't give co-sleeping a second thought. Jack slept with us for a while too. It was amazing having the whole family curled up together – even if I got about four inches of the bed allocated to me and slept in some awkward positions.

I tell pregnant women to do what works for them and their families. Everything is so finite with babies – there are only small for such a short period of time and they move through stages quickly. I now look back on those early days with a fondness that I would not have had if the kids had been sleeping alone in their rooms. Do what works best for you and if you decide to co-sleep, don't feel guilty or beat yourself up about it. Just do it as safely as possible.

AUTHOR'S NOTE: It is easy for the media to scare women into making decisions that go against their instinct. Babies are fluid and continually go through stages. Blake researched the right solution for her family and made it as safe as possible.

CHAPTER 8

APPRECIATE CHANGING FEEDING, SLEEPING & GROWTH PATTERNS (PARTNER*)

BREASTFEEDING DOESN'T HAVE TO SUCK if you can appreciate and adapt to the baby's changing feeding and sleeping patterns. Babies' needs change constantly as they grow and life gets easier in stages as you learn the new normal.

A lot of the first three months of having a new baby involves learning curves. Just when you think you can't take it anymore, whatever was causing hardship changes. Both physically and mentally the mother is recovering AND nurturing a newborn. It is hard work.

Knowing ahead of time that your baby's patterns and schedules will change will help you through the rough times. Believe me, there will be a time (in about 13 years) when you won't be able to get your child out of bed and he will be able to feed himself without you being within his sight. In the meantime, learn about the adjustments that babies make as they grow and how the breast adapts.

NOTE CHANGING SUCK AND SWALLOW PATTERNS

When a baby first latches, she usually sucks vigorously to stimulate the milk ejection reflex (let down). Once milk lets down, the baby tends to slow down into a pattern of sucking and swallowing. Many pumps have an adjustable speed and suction control in order to allow you to mimic the baby's suck pattern.

In the early stages of breastfeeding, babies often have bursts of continuous sucking before they swallow. Ten or more sucks in a row followed by swallowing would not be uncommon. This is probably due to the baby collecting small drops of colostrum into a mouthful before swallowing.

When breast milk dilutes and increases in volume (*comes in*) somewhere around day 3-8, babies form a shorter suck to swallow ratio – probably because they have more milk in the mouth faster. Suck-swallow (1:1) or suck suck-swallow (2:1) or suck suck suck-swallow (3:1) followed by breathing are all normal patterns. A baby may also pause for 3-5 seconds before they begin sucking again.

When the pause between bursts of sucking increases and the suck ratio slows, the baby is getting **full and/or tired**. If you want to encourage the baby to take a few more sucks, **raise their little baby arm up in the air from the hand or wrist and gently kiss it or rub it on your cheek**. This *priming of the pump (pictured)* often awakens them enough to take just a little bit more.

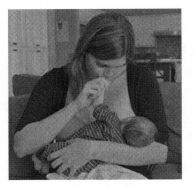

Occasionally a baby will suck but not swallow! This means that the mother thinks the baby is receiving breastmilk because he is sucking during a feed but not *transferring* (swallowing) milk. This can be highly frustrating because the baby appears to be feeding a lot but not gaining weight. Listen for the **kah kah** noise that a baby makes when they have milk in their mouth. If in doubt that the baby is actually swallowing, contact a lactation consultant. She will observe the baby's positioning, latch, jaw, mouth seal, angle of mouth opening, and rhythm (suck swallow ratio) to see where the problem lies.

EXPECT THE NUMBER OF DAILY FEEDS TO CHANGE

The recommendation for how often a baby should be fed in order to satisfy proper growth has varied dramatically over the years. In the 1960s, babies were brought to their mothers for feeding (or bottle fed in the nursery) every four hours. Eventually the recommendation changed to every three hours. Most books today recommend a newborn should be fed 8-12 times in 24 hours. Finally, evidence based research suggests that *10 or more in 24* (10 or more feeds in a 24 hours period) is currently the most adequate number of feeds in the first *two weeks* for the baby to regain his birth weight and avoid or reduce jaundice.

When I talk about *10 or more in 24* in class, I can see mothers pupils dilate. Ten feeds a day is tiring and restrictive. If a feed lasts half an hour, you are probably starting a new feed 90-120 minutes after the last one. Just remember that ten feeds a day is the best option for avoiding the need to supplement with artificial baby milk in the early days. Once the baby has regained his or her birthweight, you can adjust the feeding schedule.

> ➤ At 2-6 weeks, it is likely that the baby is feeding 7-8+ times in 24 hours.
> ➤ At 6-10 weeks, it is likely that the baby is feeding 6+ times in 24 hours.
> ➤ At 10 weeks-5 months, it is likely that the baby is feeding 5+ times in 24 hours.

> At 5-6 months, it is likely that the baby is feeding 4+ times in 24 hours.

When solid food is introduced at 6 months, it is likely that the baby will breastfeed feed 3+ times in 24 hours.

BUT ALL BABIES DIFFER and do not stick to hard and fast rules! Do you drink when you are not thirsty? Do you reach for a glass of lemonade if you are bored? Does sucking on something help to pacify you? Breastfed babies often go to the breast for reasons other than hunger. The numbers quoted per day earlier are *food feeds and some babies snack rather than have complete meals.*

CALCULATE A BABY'S NEEDS BY WEIGHT

When you are breastfeeding a baby, you never really know how much the baby is taking in because you don't have a see-through breast! Breastfeeding is estimation. You work out when they are hungry and when they have had enough. **However if you are away from your baby and she needs to be fed pumped breastmilk,** there is a relatively simple calculation to give you an *approximation* of **how many ounces** you will need **for each day of the first month.** It is based on the guideline of a baby needing *roughly* 120 calories per kilo of weight and breastmilk containing roughly 19 calories per ounce:

1. Convert your baby's weight to kilos. 1 pound = 0.4536 k
2. Multiply the baby's (k) weight by 120 calories (if he was full-term).
3. Divide the total number of calories by 19.
4. Then divide by the average daily number of feeds.

What follows is an example of the approximate number of ounces of milk a 3 week old baby would need. He was born weighing 6lbs 6oz, lost 6 ounces in the first several days and then regained his birthweight by day 11 (6lbs 6 oz.). After that he gained roughly an ounce a day. At 3 weeks (day 21), he is now 7lbs and feeding 8 times per day. His mother is going back to work and wants to know how much to pump for him on a daily basis.

EXAMPLE: 3 Week Old Baby (now weighing 7lbs)

1. A 3 week old baby weighing 7lb is equal to 3.2 kilos. *(Step 1 7lb x 0.4536 kg=3.2K)*.
2. Multiplying the kilo weight by 120 gives you **381** calories needed per day. *(Step 2 = 3.2 x 120)*
3. If breastmilk (2-6 wks. postpartum) contains an average of **19** calories per ounce, the baby would need roughly **20 ounces per day** *(Step 3 - 381 ÷ 19=20)*
4. If you divide 20 ounces by **8 feeds per 24 hr day**, then you'd be aiming for roughly **2.5 ounces (74 ml) per feed**. If the baby was feeding more or less times per day, you would need to adjust amounts accordingly.

Of the eight feeds over 24 hours, let's say the mother is able to breast feed the baby for four of them when she is home. In that case she'd be pumping roughly four times while she is away from the baby and aiming for 2.5 – 3oz each time she pumped (total from both breasts). That would give her 10oz-12oz to bring home with her for the next day.

STEADY THE COURSE IN MONTHS 1-6

As the months carry on, the baby should continue to gain weight but will probably do so at a *slightly* slower pace. His or her daily total milk intake in ounces will probably be split over fewer feeds. The baby may feed less times per day but is getting the same (or more) amount overall. As the baby grows, he or she also becomes more efficient at removing milk from the breast faster.

Remember that weight gain is an individual thing and that babies that are breastfed tend to grow and put on more weight in the first 2-3 months of life than babies who are fed with artificial baby milk/formula. **However in months 3-12, breastfed babies tend to lag behind the weight gain of a formula fed baby.** This lag can concern pediatricians especially if the baby falls off their growth curve. Amazing as it may seem, some doctors still use old growth charts that don't take exclusive breastfeeding into account. If your doctor recommends supplementing, ask questions of the growth chart (is it current – i.e. not pre-2006) and weight gain goals.

Expected Growth in the First Year

AGE (Mths)	Weight gain goals per Day
0-3	0.88 oz/25gm (or more)
3-6	0.81 oz/23gm (or more)
6-9	0.53 oz/15gm (or more)
9-12	0.42 oz/12gm

*A pound equals 16 oz or 454 grams.

Babies who are exclusively breastfed take an average of 25 ounces per 24 hour day but the range is anywhere from **19-30 ounces**. So a three month old drinking 25 ounces a day over 5 feeds is now having 5 ounces per feed. Depending on how much you pump per breast, you can get an idea of how often and how much you would need to pump daily to keep the baby fed the following day.

Despite the baby gaining weight and getting bigger, **the baby's milk requirement usually starts to slowly *decrease* as solid food is introduced at six months (or occasionally earlier or later)**. At that point milk starts to become a supplement to the meal instead of the main meal. We are the only mammals that continue to drink milk from our mothers once we are weaned onto solid food!

WAIT! MY BREASTS DON'T FEEL FULL ANYMORE

In the first couple weeks of having a newborn, many mothers tend to **overproduce**! This overproduction allows a woman to pump large amounts of breastmilk, leak easily and even spray milk out of the nipple and areola during let down. However it is NORMAL for production to become better regulated as the baby grows – typically around the 6-12 week mark.

Better regulation means that the breasts may feel softer and not engorge like they did when the baby was younger. **This does not mean that the mother is not producing enough**; it means the mother's body has worked out how much production is necessary and is now getting it right on a daily basis.

> **TIP**: SOFT BREASTS DO NOT USUALLY MEAN LOW MILK SUPPLY!

As babies get older, they also become more efficient at removing milk from the breast. What once took 30-40 minutes at 3 weeks old may now take 10-15 minutes at 3 months. Older babies (4 months+) are also distracted easier and may come off the breast, play and then go back on. Finally, a baby that has been sleeping well in the night may start waking again. This is more likely to be teething, sickness, sleep regression or not taking in enough during the day – not the mother's milk supply.

Bigger babies may need weaning to solid foods sooner than smaller ones – talk to your pediatrician if you believe the baby is ready for solids early. Supplementing with an extra ounce or two of breastmilk at bedtime may help the baby sleep longer. The mother's supply is often lowest around her own dinner time – which is often right before the baby's bedtime.

The worry that the mother is not producing enough can cause her to suddenly look for ways to increase her supply when, in actual fact, her supply is in harmony with the baby's needs. Some women even resort to supplementing with formula in an effort to keep the baby's appetite in check. **Remember, if the baby is gaining adequate weight and having wet and dirty diapers on a regular basis, there is nothing wrong with your milk supply. Your body has just perfected it!**

ANTICIPATE GROWTH SPURTS & *BOOB LAG*

Last year my son grew four inches. In the words of his pediatrician "that was an almighty growth spurt". Growth spurts (*also called frequency days*) traditionally occur at the 7-10 day mark, at 2-3 weeks, 4-6 weeks, 3 months, 4 months and 6 months but not all babies are traditional! Growth spurts can last 2-3 days and you usually realize your baby is in one as it starts to end! Babies will want to feed more and may be cranky during the spurt. There is also a theory that babies have changes in behavior (which could mean feeding more) as they move into a new (physical or neurological) developmental stage.

When a baby suddenly demands more milk, it can take the breast a day or so to catch up on supply. I call this **boob lag** – sort of like jet lag of the breasts. Just about the time your body catches up to the new demands, the baby often reverts back to their old habits so your breasts may take another day to recover back to their normal production – just like your sleep patterns when you cross time zones.

ADJUST TO CHANGING SLEEP PATTERNS

"How much does a baby sleep?" If you ask that question to most new parents, they would probably say 'not enough'. Interestingly newborns sleep a lot - roughly 16+ hours a day and when they are not sleeping, they are eating! The main problem for most parents is that babies sleep in small chunks and then need to be fed, burped, changed and comforted a lot – not always in that order.

Here is a chart of *general sleep requirements in the first year*. <u>Please remember that this is a guide and that not all babies need the same amount of sleep (now and forever)</u>. It can be useful to keep a diary to note (changing) patterns.

Age (months)	Total # of hours sleep (in 24)
0-1	16-17
1-2	15-16
2-3	14.5-15
3-4	14.5-15
4-6	15
6-12	14.5-15

For the first month or more, you should expect to be feeding in the night (between 11pm – 6am) two to three times. I know that seems scary but it is one of those things that mothers get used to doing. I compare the first three months of having a newborn like walking through a long dark tunnel. You know there is an end (to the relentless night waking and tiredness) but you just can't see it yet.

As babies stomachs grow, they take more at a feed, feed less frequently, are awake a bit longer overall and sleep longer in between feeds at night. Somewhere between **6-12 weeks**, the baby will probably start sleeping a longer stretch (4-6 hours continuously) in the night and this is considered *'sleeping through'*. Between **4-8 months (and depending on when you wean to solid foods)**, many babies will sleep for 10-12 hours at night. When your baby starts sleeping for 10-12 straight hours, you will not know what to do with yourself – but I'm sure you'll find things to do!

Breastmilk is not as high in calories as artificial baby milk/formula and so breastfed babies may wake more often for feeding at night until solid food is introduced.

AM I AWAKE OR ASLEEP?

Babies have **six** different states of consciousness - quiet sleep, active sleep, drowsy, quiet alert, active alert and crying. Sometimes it is hard to tell them apart – especially in the early days. The 'drowsy' state is transitional because the baby is drowsy both waking up from and going into sleep.

Around month four, many babies appear to regress in their sleeping habits, waking easier and more often. It is not uncommon for a baby who has been sleeping soundly for 5 solid hours to now be waking up every two or three. This regression is often because the four month old baby is in the **active** sleep cycle for longer and is woken easier than a newborn that falls into the **quiet** sleep state quickly.

Babies (like adults) fluctuate between quiet and active sleep and often awaken for a few seconds as they transition. Most go back to sleep

CHARACTERISTICS	BEHAVIORS
Quiet Sleep No rapid eye movement under lid Very still with lack of movement Can startle – 'Moro Reflex' Has bursts of sucking even though asleep	Very difficult to wake and/or feed If awoken, falls back to sleep easily Alternates between Quiet and Active Sleep (below)
Active Sleep Rapid eye movement often apparent Breathing may be irregular May smile or make facial expressions More responsive to noise	Slightly easier to wake Often confused with being awake Difficult to feed
Drowsy (Transitional State) In between Sleep and Alert (awake) or Alert and Sleep hence 'transitional' "7 mile stare" Eyes glazed over Delay in responding to stimuli Just waking up or starting to slow down	Baby is starting to wake up from OR go into active or quiet sleep If baby has been asleep, may go back to quiet or active sleep if left alone Can see, hear and track things Good time to start getting ready to feed (get a drink, etc.) if baby is waking
Quiet Alert Awake, attentive but relatively still Responsive	Great time to talk to, interact with or feed the baby Try slowly sticking your tongue out & watch for mimicking.
Active Alert Peak of movement Make noises Sometimes get fussy	Babies feed well in this stage Stretch and kick Facial movements
Crying Facial sadness or anger Cries Breathes irregularly	No longer needs stimulation May try to console self or need consoling May need change

Six States of Consciousness n Newborns

quickly but others wake up more fully. If the baby has always been rocked, cuddled or held until they were in the quiet sleep state, he or she has probably not learned how to self soothe back to sleep and they will cry out for help. It takes time for a baby to learn to self-soothe and some babies need comfort and reassurance.

Most research suggests that in order to teach self-soothing, you should establish a nap or night time routine, put the baby down to sleep while still awake (in the drowsy state) and keep the sleeping/napping area dark so the baby makes an association with darkness and sleep. I think my child knew it was nap time when I pulled down her black out blind.

There are many prescriptive books that introduce strict routines or controlled crying methods to help babies sleep transition from one state to another and sleep 'through the night'. Some parents have great success with these guide books whereas others do not. If you want to try to instigate some sort of routine, you could start by waking the baby <u>at the same time every morning</u> to help establish circadian rhythms and feeding times.

A study published in *Early Childhood Development and Care* in 2019 found that use of parenting books was associated with increased depressive symptoms and maternal stress, alongside lower self-efficacy. Although those who found the books useful had greater well-being, the majority did not find them useful. While we can help shape children a great deal, every child is unique and may have very different requirements than what *the book* says they should.

SUMMARY:

☐Babies suck and swallow patterns can give you an idea of when they are getting full and how efficiently they are transferring milk. Raising a baby's arm is like priming the pump and often awakens their appetite.

☐As babies grow, the daily number of feeds tends to decline. The overall amount of milk they are taking daily however remains relatively steady. They just take more at fewer feeds.

☐If you are pumping and feeding from a bottle, there is a four step equation you can use to calculate the number of ounces needed per day.

☐Babies take an average of 19-30 ounces of milk per day in month 1-6. Breastfed babies tend to lag behind the weight gain of a formula fed baby in months 3-12.

☐A mother's milk supply tends to stabilize and regulate over time and her breasts may not feel or look full. That DOES NOT mean her supply is low; it means her body has adjusted to her baby's needs.

☐During a 2-3 day growth spurt a baby's feeding and sleeping requirements may increase. The breastfeeding woman's body often requires time to catch up to the new demand (*boob lag*).

☐Baby's sleep patterns vary enormously but most babies sleep an average of 15 hours a day in months 1-6. Strict routines work for some parents but cause stress and depression for others. Eventually babies will fall into regular patterns of sleeping and eating more in line with their family's schedule.

☐Babies cycle through six states of consciousness – quiet sleep, active sleep, drowsy, quiet alert, active alert and crying. It is impossible to feed a baby in the quiet sleep state. A change in sleep patterns around month 3-4 means that babies who have always been put down asleep may not know how to self soothe. Putting a baby down when drowsy is a useful start to helping the baby learn to get to sleep by themselves.

LIFE THROWS YOU A FRISBEE - CAROLINA'S STORY

What I initially thought were painful Braxton Hicks contractions started on the morning of June 6th but then stopped. They started again around 4pm. At 11pm I took a shower and thought 'This is it!' I woke my husband at 1am (now June 7th) and went to the hospital only to be told I was "only 1-2 cms" and, after an hour of walking around with no change, went home. Once back home, labor kicked off again quickly. I had an urge to push which made me feel out of control. After the 3rd pushing contraction, my water broke. We thought perhaps the baby was about to be born so my husband called the hospital who told him to call 911 (emergency). The next thing I know, loads of 1st responders were in my house to take me to the nearest hospital (which was not the hospital where I was registered to give birth!).

Upon arrival at the 2nd hospital, I was at measured at 5 cm and in a great deal of pain. They refused to give me an epidural until I had some tests and an IV for fluids. At 2 pm, I was measuring 7cm but I then stalled completely for the next 6 hours. The baby was thought to be posterior (back to back) and nothing – not even a peanut ball – could coax her out of that position. By this point my hips were hurting, my cervix was swollen, I had a fever and was shaking (teeth rattling) so a decision was taken to move to Cesarean. I was so exhausted by this point – it was like having a Frisbee or two thrown at you without warning.

During the cesarean, I could pinpoint where they were cutting me so they briefly put me to sleep. I woke up right before she was born and got to hear her cry. At that point, everything changed. Melania's cry made me realize that it was all worth it but I was thankful that labor was over! Without warning, they took her to the NICU where she would stay for the next three days. She was born at 9.10 pm and I didn't get to see her until 11pm. They checked me for infection for the next two days but I was cleared and discharged.

Unfortunately, the NICU fed my baby formula for the first day (2 oz. at each feeding). Two ounces seemed far too much for a newborn's tiny stomach but there was no discussion. I was asked if I wanted to breastfeed her (which I did) but there was no one to help me. The baby and I struggled with latching and it was very painful. Then I was informed that she "wasn't getting anything" from me so I had to give her formula again.

Later that day, I went to the NICU again – this time with a lactation consultant. She helped me use a supplemental nursing system (SNS) at the breast. She also helped with me with the nipple damage by introducing me to breast shells, lanolin and using my own colostrum on the wound. I even managed to pump a drop or two of colostrum which was fed to the baby! I took Melania home on Day 4 armed with a nipple shield. My mother and sister told me not to use the shield; they said that 'breastfeeding always hurts!' I beg to differ.

I tried breastfeeding without the nipple shield several times but it was just too painful. At three months I went to see the lactation consultant again. She taught me the 'flipple' which allowed a latch without pain. I was SO EXCITED. After that, it was easy to tell when the baby was latched well or not. I also used the Haakaa every feed to help improve supply but I learned how quickly the baby could start to prefer the easy drip of breastmilk from a bottle over the harder work of pulling it out of the breast. Eventually I got her back to the breast 100% by ditching the nipple shield.

In the end, I had months of 'frisbees' (and they still keep coming!). The birth in a different hospital, an unplanned C-Section, 4 days in the NICU, formula, SNS and nipple shields to name a few. But WE DID IT and are still breastfeeding strong at 8 months!! I truly believe the key to successful breastfeeding is consistency, persistence and a good latch.

AUTHOR'S NOTE: During Carolina's labor, she felt an early urge to push which threw her into a panic. This urge could have been caused by the baby making a ¼ turn and descending into the pelvis around 5 cm. It's unfortunate that she ended up in a hospital that was foreign to her – it's not surprising that the stress caused her adrenaline to pump and labor to stall.

With no lactation expertise to help Carolina hand express or support the first few latches, she had little choice but to give the baby formula in the NICU. Thankfully Carolina eventually found help from a lactation consultant and a nipple shield. She told me that the 'flipple' changed her life because she was able to feed pain-free with this technique.

Overall, Carolina's persistence and motivation turned a dreadful start into a fulfilling and life altering experience. She continues to have parenting 'frisbees' (sleep regression, teething, weaning, etc.) thrown at her but now she has got very good at researching solutions and throwing that Frisbee right back from where it came.

CHAPTER 9

CREATE A DEPENDABLE MILK SUPPLY

BREASTFEEDING DOESN'T HAVE TO SUCK *if you can create a reliable and plentiful milk supply.*

The number one reason that women give up breastfeeding is the **perception that they are not manufacturing an adequate supply of breastmilk ("I don't have enough")**. Sometimes this assumption is based on the sudden increase in demand after a night of cluster feeding at the 72 hour mark (especially if milk is delayed due to labor meds or water retention) or during a growth spurt (often the first one hitting around 10 days – 2 weeks). Sometimes it is based on the woman's inability to pump the same amount as before or when she no longer wakes up engorged. Regardless of the reason for doubt, the supply is *almost* always ample.

Remember, if the baby is gaining weight and having regular wet and dirty diapers, your supply is perfect. However, there are ways to get your supply off to a good start, maintain it or increase it if your care provider diagnoses you 'clinically low'.

TICK THE BOXES?

Before we look at possible ways to improve the milk supply, what follows is a *summary* of some of the things that could be depleting or reducing a milk supply. If you can answer YES to any of the questions, your milk supply may be low due to that reason. It is often easier to improve or correct the depletion rather than trying to artificially increase your supply with a supplement or excessive pumping.

WHAT'S REDUCING MY MILK SUPPLY?

- ☐ Am I only partially emptying the breast or timing feedings too rigorously?
- ☐ Is the baby getting a bottle a lot (reducing skin to skin and breast stimulation)?
- ☐ Am I anemic or experiencing low thyroid function?
- ☐ Am I ingesting more than 300 mcg of caffeine (coffee, energy drinks, etc.) per day?
- ☐ Am I ingesting more than 300 mcg of theobromine (dark chocolate) per day?
- ☐ Am I taking a prenatal vitamin instead of a postnatal one?
- ☐ Am I using a lot of herbs (sage, parsley, thyme, oregano)?
- ☐ Am I using/eating a lot of menthol mints, spearmint or peppermint (ex. tea, candies)
- ☐ Is the baby taking less because of weaning to solids?
- ☐ Am I not getting enough Vitamin A, C, E and Choline?
- ☐ Am I not eating enough Calories (>2200 kcals) and Carbohydrates (210g+) per day?
- ☐ Am I drinking too much alcohol?
- ☐ Am I still using a nipple shield?
- ☐ Am I exercising too much?
- ☐ Is the baby using a pacifier before or in between feeds?
- ☐ Am I smoking more than 20 cigarettes a day or vaping?
- ☐ Am I using any Cannabis Based Derivatives?
- ☐ Am I using any allergy or cold remedies (ex. Benadryl, Sudafed)
- ☐ Am I using Birth control (including the Depo injection) before 6 weeks postpartum?
- ☐ Am I using birth control pills containing estrogen?
- ☐ Has my period started again?
- ☐ Am I pregnant again?

DRINK TO THIRST & EAT HEALTHY

Many women believe that they must up their intake of fluids in order to breastfeed successfully. In fact, the current recommendation for lactating mothers is to **'drink to thirst'** instead of drinking a prescribed amount of water on a daily basis. While normal hydration is important for the mother's own *health*, **and she may be more thirsty when breastfeeding**, there is no magic number of ounces you should drink per day. Drink when you are thirsty and do not become dehydrated.

Also, realize that while 1000 mg per day of calcium is essential, **you do not need to drink cow's milk to make breastmilk**. We are the only mammals who drink other mammal's milk and in my house I refer to cheese and butter as *processed cow's hindmilk*! Also, the most common allergen that affects a baby's digestion through your breastmilk is one or both of the milk proteins called casein and whey. You can get plenty of calcium from broccoli, leafy greens, almonds, almond milk, tahini, tofu and beans to name a few. But if you do drink cow's milk, the current recommendation is to drink the low-fat or skim variety.

Women often ask me what they should eat when they are breastfeeding. The short answer is to **eat a healthy balanced diet** (check out www.choosemyplate.gov for ideas). It takes energy to make breastmilk, recover from illness and change diapers in the middle of the night and different parts of your body compete for the energy from the foods you eat. A breastfeeding woman eating a well-balanced diet will be healthier overall and that will keep the baby healthier too.

What you eat can also affect the baby longer term. Evidence continues to pile up about the Western diet being overly stacked with unhealthy processes including the amount of **unhealthy fats and**

added sugar. It is fair to say that women who have a healthy diet are sending a better quality of fat through their breastmilk. If you are eating a fast-food cheeseburger, so is your baby.

There is also a recent study that positively correlates excess weight gain in the baby (and potentially later in life) with **fructose** in the mother's diet. Fructose is a popular sweetener added to foods and drinks to make them taste or look better. When you combine fructose with glucose, you get high-fructose corn syrup – another common ingredient in the Western diet. It is no surprise that fructose leaking into breast milk could have negative consequences. In adults, excessive consumption of fructose is linked to insulin resistance, obesity, elevated LDL cholesterol and triglycerides potentially leading to diabetes and heart disease.

Have a look at the chart comparing recommendations on the daily intake of various vitamins and minerals for the non-pregnant, pregnant and breastfeeding woman to see where you can adjust your diet.

	NON-PREGNANT	PREGNANT	BREASTFEEDING
Energy (calories/day)	2400	2500-2700	2700-2800
Carbohydrates ((g/day)	130	175	210
Protein	46	71	71
Fat (% of total calories)	20-35%	20-35%	20-35%
Iron (mg/day)	18	27	9
Calcium (mg/day)	1000	1000	1000
Iodine (mcg/day)	150	220	290
Magnesium (mg/day)	320	350-360	310-320
Vitamin A (mcg/day)	700	770	1300
Vitamin D (mcg/day)	5	5	5
Vitamin C (mg/day)	75	85	120
Vitamin E (mg/day)	15	15	19
Folate (mcg/day)	400	600	500
Choline (mg/day)	425	450	550

In this chart, note the most drastic changes in the recommended daily allowance (RDA) from pregnancy to breastfeeding: the RDA of iron decreases by two-thirds, the RDA of Iodine (which many get from salt) increases by 32%, the RDA of Vitamin A increases 69%, Vitamin C and E increase by 41% and 27% respectively. Finally, choline intake is recommended to increase by 22%. If you are not sure how to read food labels, check out **www.fda.gov** (Food/Labeling Nutrition).

AVOID AVOID AVOID

There are a few foods that you should avoid when breastfeeding. It is best to avoid **fish containing mercury** (ex. Shark, swordfish, tilefish, king mackerel) due to the harm the mercury could do to the baby's developing nervous system. You should also limit white canned tuna to 6 oz. or less per week. For those who love sushi, find out what kind of fish is being used to see if you can indulge – most sushi is safe.

There are a few common herbs that – if used in abundance – could hinder your supply of breastmilk. A pinch while cooking is not a worry but used in larger quantities, the following common herbs may help deplete or reduce a fickle milk supply: **Oregano, Thyme, Sage and Parsley**. In addition, your supply of breastmilk can be particularly sensitive to **spearmint, peppermint and menthol**.

LIMIT TOXIN INTAKE

There are many foods that are frowned upon or women are told to exclude during pregnancy but with breastfeeding, you have more gastro-freedom. When I suggest that you measure *toxin intake*, I mean substances like alcohol, chocolate and coffee (caffeine). Women are often under the impression that they can have none of these things and it can make breastfeeding seem a bit like a punishment. Just be wise by monitoring and limiting your intake.

The American Academy of Pediatrics' current recommendation for caffeine intake is up to 300 mg of caffeine per day if the baby was healthy and full term. At Starbucks, you'd get about 300mg in just one Venti Caffe Americano® but only half that in a Grande or Venti Caffe Latte®, Grande Carmel Macchiato® or Expresso. There are now quite a few apps which can tell you the amount of caffeine in your drink depending on size and brand. There are also many websites that do the same including **www.caffeineinformer.com**.

At home, 300mg is roughly two average cups of instant coffee or tea. Also, beware of **energy drinks** and other sources of caffeine like **sodas/pop**. A 16 oz. can of Monster Energy® drink has 160mg of caffeine. Just like with people, caffeine can have no effect or a dramatic effect on the baby as it passes into him or her through the

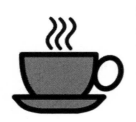 mother's breastmilk. Look for signs of fussiness or excessive wakefulness that might signal your baby is being affected and reduce your intake accordingly.

Stressed spelled backwards is **desserts** and sometimes life is vastly improved with a little *chocolate*. However chocolate should also be monitored because of a potential toxin called **theobromine**. This close relative to caffeine has almost identical effects on a baby if a large amount is consumed and should be limited to 300mg per day. An ***ounce of milk chocolate*** contains approximately 6mg of theobromine but ***dark chocolate*** is roughly 10 times that of milk chocolate – 60mg per ounce. So if you had two grande lattes from Starbucks (300 mg of caffeine) and 5 oz. of dark chocolate, (300mg of theobromine), you might find the baby reacting negatively.

While it is unlikely that most people would eat large amounts of dark chocolate in bar form, it can be found in chocolate sauces, chocolate chips and dark chocolate desserts. As a general rule, the darker and more expensive the chocolate, the more theobromine that is potentially present (theobromine is in the more expensive cocoa solid which gives chocolate the deeper brown color). White chocolate has no theobromine in it so it is an alternative with no theobromine downside. As with caffeine, monitor the baby for signs of fussiness or excessive wakefulness and alter your intake as needed.

Drinking alcohol is one of the most emotive subjects I have ever come across. Research indicates that babies that are exposed to alcohol in breastmilk tend to take less and have fragmented sleep. However breastfeeding guru Dr Jack Newman feels that we shouldn't completely abstain but rather be careful:

"Reasonable alcohol intake should not be discouraged at all. As is the case with most drugs, very little alcohol comes out in the milk. The mother can take some alcohol and continue breastfeeding as she normally does. Prohibiting alcohol is another way we make life unnecessarily restrictive for nursing mothers."

The key words in that statement are 'reasonable' and 'some'. A glass of wine with dinner is far different than binge drinking for six hours. I once heard a midwife say "if you shouldn't be driving, you shouldn't be feeding a baby" and that is a liberal rule of thumb. To be on the cautious side, you could breastfeed the baby before drinking any alcohol and make sure the baby is asleep before having an alcoholic drink. According to Motherisk in Toronto, an average height woman who weighs 68K/150lbs will require 2 hours 14 minutes to metabolize and clear alcohol in her breastmilk from one average drink.

If you can still feel the effect of alcohol, you can feed the baby stored milk from previous pumping sessions while you 'pump and dump' to keep up your supply. Another useful idea is to eat food while drinking alcohol so alcohol absorption is lessened. Finally, milk 'strips' for testing the alcohol content are now on the market and can *possibly* take the guess work out of *'safe'* alcohol content although some are more efficient than others.

The benefits of a **cigarette smoking** mother breastfeeding her baby far outweigh the risks of a cigarette smoking mother **not** breastfeeding her baby. However protecting the baby from 2nd hand smoke is essential. The best way to protect a baby is to smoke outside or in another room with an extra layer of clothing on. Then, before picking up or feeding the baby, remove the extra layer of clothing that you wore when smoking and wash your hands. And of course quit if at all possible.

We may have only seen the tip of the iceberg so far with marijuana use by the mother and the effects on a breastfed baby. Despite the harmless reputation of **marijuana and cannabinoids (CBDs),** some studies suggest it can disable your ability to make enough milk, cause undue sleepiness in the baby, alter developing brain cells and build up THC in breastmilk (which attaches to fat). Mothers can test positive for up to two weeks after use and babies can test positive for as long as three weeks! No study that I have seen states any positive physiological outcome for marijuana users who breastfeed and marijuana may negatively affect the mother's mental state and ability to care for herself and the baby.

If you are unable to stop smoking or ingesting marijuana, then I would try to decrease your usage as much as possible and shield your baby from second hand smoke as mentioned earlier (by keeping the baby in a separate room when smoking, washing your hands and changing the top layer of your clothes before holding and feeding them). Until further research and various regulatory bodies give recommendations, it is suggested that the breastfeeding mother stays as far away from cannabis as possible.

WHAT ELSE COULD DISRUPT SUPPLY?

I can't tell you the number of women who have disrupted their milk supply (or caused interesting diapers) by taking a medication without realizing the potential effect it could have. Check the label of **any**

supplements or medications (prescribed or over-the-counter) before taking them. A simple cold medicine or allergy reliever (like **Sudafed or Benadryl**) could affect a fragile milk supply. If it dries up your sinuses, it could dry up other parts too! Remember to check LactMed before taking a medication to decide it if is safe with breastfeeding: **(https://www.toxnet.nlm.nih.gov).**

Taking **prenatal vitamins or iron** in the postnatal period is often recommended by a care provider but not supported by evidence based research. Although there is no current study that suggests prenatal vitamins affect milk supply, I've spoken to countless mothers who noticed an increase when they stopped taking them. You can try your own experiment – stop taking them for a few days and see if it makes a difference or replace your prenatal vitamin with a postnatal one.

Ovulation, menstruation and birth control pills containing estrogen can also reduce or affect your supply. **Cutting calories** below 2200 per day, **over exercising**, a **lack of rest** and **over pumping** can also reduce milk supply. Remember that most actions have reactions and those reactions can sometimes result in a lower milk supply!

IMPROVE YOUR SUPPLY BY HAND

Up to this point, we have been discussing things that could disrupt or decrease your milk supply. If you have gone through 'What's Reducing My Milk Supply' list without being able to tick any boxes or improve upon any of those situations, the rest of the chapter is dedicated to various ways of increasing your supply.

One of the oldest tricks in the book is to gently massage the breast before and during a feed (or pumping session). This is thought to awaken the ducts. Gently massage all around the visible part of the breast in small circles with your fingertips or knuckles. Some women prefer using an electric toothbrush, warm washcloth or compress to help with let down while others do a small amount of gentle shaking of the breast (the milk shake!) in order to assist let down and production. There are also a number of battery powered breast massagers on the market that both heat and massage the area with little effort.

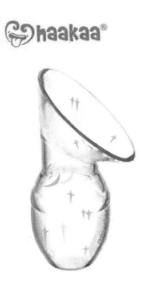

Another (and relatively new) device for increasing milk supply is a *passive* silicone pump. Looking a bit like a tiny transparent bottle with a tuba-like opening, it is attached to the breast by squeezing air out of the bottom and suctioning it onto the 2nd breast. The suction encourages drops of milk from the breast. Many women are able to drip an ounce or more during a feed which can be used another time when supply is low.

One of the first 'catchers' of this type was developed by a woman from New Zealand and named the HaaKaa® - although there are many brands that do the same thing on the market. By dripping out an extra ounce during a feed, your body will then maintain or increase milk supply accordingly.

PUMP IT UP!

In order to increase supply, many women begin pumping almost immediately. In my opinion, this makes the USA a nation of **'over-pumpers'**. A lot of women pump without really thinking about the dependency they are creating. Removing milk with a pump one day causes the body to make a little more the next day – thereby increasing supply. Then, if the baby then takes the extra you produce the next day, the supply should stabilize at the higher level. But if the baby does not take the extra you've created, you will have more milk than you need and you will have to pump to avoid engorgement!

Pumping then becomes a daily habit without a real benefit and creates a vicious circle of **pumping exhaustion, possible clogged ducts and even mastitis. Pumping is useful if** the baby is unable to latch, you are building a stockpile of milk for your absence or for use later in the day or night when you are exhausted and your milk-making abilities may be less efficient. But if you are pumping to increase supply, you should be doing it short term – maybe once every other day for a few days. It would be wise to let your baby and body establish your milk supply requirements for the first several weeks before going near a pump!

If you do pump, understand that the amount of milk a woman can pump varies greatly – and does not always have a direct correlation to her milk supply. For example, some women cannot coerce any milk out of the breast with a pump if the mother cannot see, hear or smell the baby - while other mothers can pump 5 oz. alone in the car in traffic. Most women pump an average of 1-3 oz. total during a session. Remember that in order to let down, the body needs to release oxytocin and that can be difficult in a stressful environment. You are not a failure if you can't pump as much as someone else – it is not a competition. The breasts were designed to be pumped by the baby.

There is also no right or wrong time to pump but many women feel that pumping once in the morning – either before or one hour after the baby's first feed - works best because they have more energy. The right time for you to pump is when you feel awake and relaxed and that can be different for different women. If you were pumping at work, you would aim to pump the same time your baby would have breastfed.

DAY		MINUTES OF PUMPING	notes as needed about the session (power pumping, skin-to-skin, etc.)	OUNCES OF MILK OBTAINED	
DATE	TIME			LEFT breast	RIGHT breast
	AM / PM	min.		oz.	oz.
	AM / PM	min.		oz.	oz.
	AM / PM	min.		oz.	oz.
	AM / PM	min.		oz.	oz.
	AM / PM	min.		oz.	oz.
	AM / PM	min.		oz.	oz.
	AM / PM	min.		oz.	oz.
	AM / PM	min.		oz.	oz.

A pumping log can be useful

You may consider keeping a log of pumping dates, times and ounces. See Chapter 12 for more information on effective pumping technique and equipment.

TRY HERBS TO IMPROVE SUPPLY

Women often turn to the health food store to improve milk supply and there are several non-prescription supplements that promise to improve prolactin manufacture and release. Many of the following suggestions **lack evidence based research** studies on effectiveness but anecdotally, many women have varying degrees of success. *You should always consider any risks of these potential solutions.*

Goat's Rue (aka French Lilac, French Honeysuckle) is a plant native to the Middle East. In 1873, a dairy farmer documented an improved milk supply in his cows after they grazed on goat's rue and it has been used as a **galactagogue** (milk supply improver) ever since. It is available as dried leaves (add 1 tsp leaves to 1 cup boiling water for 15 minute infusion and drink 1 cup twice a day), drops (2-4 ml, 2-3 times per day) or capsules. Goat's Rue may also increase breast tissue although it is not understood exactly how. *Beware that Goat's Rue can reduce blood sugar levels, cause sweating and increase frequency of trips to the toilet (urinating) because it is a diuretic.*

Fenugreek is the go-to choice for many women. The leaves and seeds of this plant are cultivated globally and used in cooking – especially curries. The herb can be purchased in drops (preferable for many), capsules or leaves (for steeping in tea). The recommended dosage is 2-4 (500mg) capsules a day or two full droppers 2-3 times per day. If you try Fenugreek, start out at a lower dose and then increase slightly over the next several days. If you do not see any change, perhaps try something else. This herb is meant to be used for a ***short duration***.

There are also ***risks to using Fenugreek***. It is in the same family as peanuts and so those with a *peanut allergy* should take note. It can also lower *blood sugar levels* which may be useful if you are diabetic but could be harmful if your blood sugar is often low. Some women report *stomach problems and upset*. Many women also report a *maple syrup smell* in their urine, irregular menstrual cycles and a *trigger for migraines*. **Finally, do not use if there is any chance you may be pregnant or are trying to get pregnant.**

Blessed Thistle is another popular choice for increasing milk supply. Do not confuse it with *milk thistle* which is in the same family. Dosage varies but 3-4 capsules three times per days or 10-20 drops (2ml) 2-4 times per day seems to work for many women. Ragweed allergy sufferers should beware of occasional adverse reactions.

The polysaccharides from **Barley** have also been shown to improve milk supply. While barley is the main ingredient in beer, non-alcoholic beer has the same effect without the ethanol from alcohol.

Barley cereals, soups and cookies are also popular choices. Some women have success increasing supply by drinking **oat milk**.

Some products like Mother's Milk® tea contain several prolactin inducing ingredients in smaller doses and may be worth a try. **Fennel, marshmallow, the Filipino plant Malunggay** (Moringa) and **alfalfa** (medicago sativa) are all popular in various parts of the world for improving milk supply. As with any drug, consider how these may interact with anything else you are eating or drinking.

TALK TO YOUR DOCTOR

If a Lactation Consultant or Doctor diagnoses your milk supply as clinically low, you may be prescribed a 'dopamine inhibitor' to increase prolactin levels for a short period of time. In the USA, Reglan (Metoclopramide) is usually the first choice. One of the major drawbacks (side effects) of Reglan however is the possibility of serious depression setting in after a few weeks. Let your care provider guide you on usage and dosage.

Another potential problem solver is Domperidone (Motilium). However Domperidone is not approved by its manufacturer for increasing milk supply (although this seems to be a well-documented side effect) and is not currently available in the USA. Like any drug, it has risks to the mother *including abdominal cramps, break through bleeding and dry mouth.* Women who take the drug longer term can experience *anxiety, sleeplessness and loss of appetite.*

TIP: Remember, if the baby is gaining weight and having regular wet and dirty diapers, your supply is perfect!

SUMMARY:

☐Breastfeeding women should drink to thirst. There is no need to drink a prescribed amount of water or fluids. There is also no need to drink (cow's) milk in order to make human milk.

☐The nutritional requirements of a breastfeeding mother are different than those of a pregnant one. Eating a healthy balanced diet provides energy. Consuming less than an average of 2200 calories per day can reduce supply.

☐Many toxins can be consumed while breastfeeding but amounts should be monitored and limited.

☐The current recommendation for caffeine and theobromine (in dark chocolate) is 300 mg a day or less.

☐Alcohol is metabolized faster with food. Feeding the baby before drinking alcohol and letting it metabolize is probably the safest way to have an alcoholic drink and breastfeed.

☐Using marijuana and cannabis based derivatives during breastfeeding has an ever growing list of risks.

☐Consider the effect any medications or supplements may have on breast milk creation. Birth control pills with estrogen have an effect on supply. Taking pre-natal vitamins during breastfeeding is not evidence based and may affect milk supply; consider a postnatal vitamin instead. If in doubt, consult the Lactmed database.

☐Milk production is a supply and demand process. One of the easy and natural ways to improve supply is to hand express or pump once a day after you feel breastfeeding is established. This tells the brain to make more milk tomorrow because demand has risen.

☐Massage, warmth, gentle shaking and attaching a passive pump to the breast are all ways to awaken ducts and improve let down which can in turn improve supply.

☐Natural supplements that may help improve milk supply include Goat's Rue, Fenugreek, Barley and Blessed Thistle.

☐For a true clinical diagnosis of low supply, a care provider may prescribe Reglan (USA) or Domperidone short term. The benefits, risks and alternatives for any drug should be discussed with your Care Provider.

A CHANGE IN PLANS – MELISSA'S JOURNEY

I really wanted a natural birth, but after an induction (due to pre-eclampsia and HELLP Syndrome) which ended in a Cesarean Section, there didn't seem to be anything natural about it. Happily though, my baby (Owen) was born healthy and weighed in at 6 lbs. 14 oz. at birth on Sunday, February 18 at 3:46 pm.

The Lactation Consultant coached me through those first two days as I recovered from surgery. I pumped every 2-3 hours in the hospital and every 3-4 hours when I got home but I had NO VISIBLE MILK. When I tried to pump, what little came out was *steamy and gooey and impossible to collect* so I ended up giving him formula since he was losing weight. I also continued to try and get him to latch after each gooey session. He seemed pretty drugged up himself – probably due to all the medications that I endured. I had wanted breastfeeding to be an easy transition but my supply was just not there. THIS WAS NOT THE PLAN!

That first week is somewhat of a blur. I was in tears many times overcoming the trauma of surgery. My husband and I were also stressed and sleep deprived. On day six, my brother-in-law and his wife came over to help. They watched and fed the baby while Jared and I slept for four solid hours! I woke up at 1pm feeling relaxed, alert and calm so I decided to try some pumping. Like magic, my milk had come in and I was able to pump. I carried out my pumped milk bottles in the air like trophies!

The *2nd week* was a little easier. We had to leave the house for my follow up appointments. As I calmed down, Owen latched easier. I breastfed and supplemented and he continued to gain weight. In the *third week*, I felt I needed to get out and talk to other women. I went to the local Breastfeeding Support Group which helped immensely. Around *week seven*, I got a crystallized painful bleb on the nipple. I tried warm showers, massage and nursing on that side. Eventually I researched it and removed it with sterile tweezers. It hurt but healed quickly with breastmilk – which is the best Neosporin ever! Breastfeeding finally became comfortable around the *two month mark*. At one point early on we thought Owen had a lip tie but the Ears, Nose & Throat (ENT) Doctor felt it wasn't worth correcting.

In June, I went on a long awaited trip to Costa Rica with over 100 students. I would be gone for nine days. I have PCOS (polycystic ovarian syndrome) so I knew that when I pumped I was going to have either the motherlode of milk or the dry lake bed. Thankfully I had an oversupply which allowed me to freeze 6 oz. a day over four months. I left behind 98 bags of milk for my husband to feed Owen. Even though I pumped when I was away, the trip was the beginning of the end of breastfeeding.

In August I went back to work. The stress of being away from the baby, rushing to pick him up, make dinner, etc. started to affect my supply. I was still able to pump at 5am, 9am and again after school at 2pm. Then I would breastfeed him at 4.30pm and again at 8pm. I was also setting the alarm clock for 1am and pumping. I tried keeping my supply up with a number of supplements like Mother's Milk™ tea, a cold brew called Upspring Baby Milk Flow™ (which contains fenugreek and blessed thistle), capsules of Fenugreek and soy lecithin (to ward off blebs).

In September and October, I went through two hugely stressful life changing events which further contributed to a slowdown in breastfeeding. I had to fly to Iowa unexpectedly as my own mother's health was failing and quickly learned the airline's stringent requirements for traveling with breastmilk. Milk needs to be in a **solid frozen state** in order to pass through airport security as a carry-on item. Owen also had six teeth by this point and started biting! Then he contracted foot and mouth disease from daycare. The irritability of a sick teething baby added further stress. Soon after that, I stopped waking myself up at night to pump.

After all that I'd been through, I set myself a goal to carry on breastfeeding until Christmas. When we introduced solids in November, I was only getting 1.5 ounces in total at a pumping session. I continued breastfeeding before and after work and in the night if needed. My breastfeeding journey finally ended in the New Year. I lived by three rules that I learned very early in breastfeeding. First of all, feed your baby. Second, enjoy your baby. Third: don't let the 1st one get in the way of the 2nd.

Through the frustrations and setbacks, I learned that stress management and good sleep was vital to my breastfeeding success. Learning to breastfeed while side-lying helped to ease the exhaustion and made for many unforgettable snuggling memories. Yoga and self-care time became equally important in maintaining my mental stamina as I transitioned into *motherhood.*

AUTHOR'S NOTE: Melissa did an amazing job – especially considering the incredible stress of Owen's first year. I would expect a delay in her milk *coming in* due to her induction and C-Section. The sticky and gooey milk she pumped was colostrum and I'm not quite sure why the Lactation Consultant did not encourage hand expression because it is almost impossible to pump with a machine. She was wise to encourage Owen to latch even when she didn't think she had any milk – she had more than she realized.

In the weeks that followed, life threw Melissa many obstacles but she persevered. Imagine the effort that went in to pump 98 six-ounce bags! A mother's milk supply usually regulates itself by around three months and most struggle to pump as much as they once did. Melissa gave Owen the best possible start in life and it has paid off. He is a healthy, happy and active baby thanks to her fantastic nurturing.

CHAPTER 10

BE AWARE OF POTENTIAL
PROBLEMS BEFORE THEY STRIKE

BREASTFEEDING DOESN'T HAVE TO SUCK *if you can spot a problem before it becomes serious and work to correct it as soon as possible.*

This chapter examines some of the issues women and babies face and potentially how to overcome them. The biggest (and probably rarest) problem of all – the inability to breastfeed – is the one with which we will start. We will also highlight some of the biggies that cause stress and fear in mothers including colic, jaundice, D-MER, mastitis and milk digestion.

WILL THE MOTHER BE ABLE TO BREASTFEED?

Statistics are often quoted about the huge percentage of women who *should* be able to breastfeed. Many women choose not to breastfeed and that is a personal decision. But often women desperately want to breastfeed without realizing that various circumstances and situations may decrease her chances. Knowing these issues in advance allows you to expect the worst, hope for the best and realize that you are doing nothing wrong if it doesn't work out. Sometimes things are out of your control.

Perhaps the most common question I get asked in class is whether **breast surgery** or **nipple piercing** can alter milk production or reduce the ability to breastfeed. The answer is maybe but probably not! Problems are more likely to occur with **breast reduction** because breast tissue (and possibly ducts) may have been removed. Let down can be affected if the nerves of the nipple and areola are damaged.

Breast enlargement can also affect breastfeeding but usually to a lesser degree. Depending on where and how the silicone/saline implant was placed, some women will experience increased swelling and tenderness. Surgeons should be well aware of the woman's future plans and usually bear this in mind when altering the breast. Speak to your care provider and breast surgeon about the details of the procedure and how it may (or may not) affect you.

Milk making is tied to hormone production and hormonal imbalances can alter the mother's ability to produce. Women who have **thyroid or adrenal issues or polycystic ovarian syndrome (PCOS)** may produce too little (or occasionally too much) milk, release milk sporadically or fail to let down at all. **Menstrual irregularities** (cycles, ovulation) and women who have conceived using **reproductive technology (IVF, etc.)** have a higher risk of a hormonal imbalance and *may* struggle making or maintaining milk.

There is a *rare* genetic disorder called **nipple atresia** where the woman's nipple has no pore openings. If this is her first baby, she would not know this beforehand. A woman with suspected atresia should be seen by a care provider immediately.

The release of the **placenta** in the 3rd stage of labor is what starts milk production. Therefore if a piece of the placenta is accidentally left behind in the uterus, the mother's body may struggle to make milk until the missing piece of the placenta passes or is surgically removed. The placenta is removed during a C-Section just like in a vaginal birth. It is the drugs used in C-Sections (or vaginal births) that can slow the influx of milk to the breast (see Chapter 3 for a refresher).

Also, as mentioned in Chapter 3, **shock brought on by severe bleeding when the placenta is delivered** (3rd Stage of labor) can result in a rare condition called Sheehan's Syndrome. The bleeding causes the mother's blood pressure to drop so low that blood fails to circulate to her pituitary gland and some or all of the cells in that gland stop working permanently. Her breasts remain soft and she may not be able to produce milk. Sadly, this is a permanent malfunction and may mean she is completely unable to breastfeed.

Whether genetic or caused by an injury to the delicate breast bud in childhood, some women suffer from breast **hypoplasia** (also known as hypomastia, micromastia or Insufficient Glandular Tissue) where the breasts don't develop to full maturity. This can be extremely troubling emotionally and physically and stifle milk production. Breast enhancement surgery can often alter the look of the breast but she may not be able to manufacture milk or breastfeed.

SHOOTING PAINS IN THE BREAST?

A good blood supply in the breast and nipple is needed in order to breastfeed well. Occasionally mothers report **a deep stabbing or burning pain deep in the breast or nipple**. It sometimes results in a white (blanched) and/or mis-shapen (lipstick looking) nipple after a feed. This is referred to as a *vasospasm* and is often triggered by a poor latch. The blood supply through the breast and to the nipple is being restricted as the blood vessels tighten and cause pain.

While the vasospasms can be caused by a bite or shallow latch, they can also be affected by cool air! Most women notice that even something as harmless as a cool breeze can kick start their pain. Existing cracks, cuts or damage to the nipple trigger vasospasms. So can anything that constricts a blood vessel like caffeine, smoking, stress and some medications (like over the counter cold remedies).

There are no foolproof solutions for vasospasms but getting help with a deeper latch, keeping warm before and during feeds and some supplements (omega fatty acids, lecithin, Vitamin B6) may help. It is best not to feed the baby while you are having a vasospasm if you can wait. Stabbing breast pains could also be Thrush (pg. 149) so visit your lactation consultant or doctor as soon as possible and tell them your symptoms so you can be treated correctly.

Some women experience shooting, stabbing or 'knife-like' pains when their milk lets down instead of the 'tingling sensation' described by others. This is usually because they have a fast flow and milk is being forced through ducts quickly which in turn causes pain. A mom recently told me she knew it was let down causing the (30 seconds of) pain because she could feel it happening on both sides at the same time. While there is not a lot you can do to avoid this, you could try a warm compress on the breast prior to feeding and a little massage to awaken the ducts. The fast let down may also become more regulated as your body adjusts.

AVOIDING PLUGGED DUCTS (BLEBS) & MASTITIS

Remember from Chapter 2 that the breast may have twenty or so ducts – so a lot of places to potentially get a **clog (plug/plugged duct)**. Ducts can develop a plug when they are not completely emptied. A block normally starts as a lump along with soreness and swelling. The first course of action most women try is either warmth (hot compresses) or cold (ice packs) 5-10 minutes before feeding or pumping. Massage can be very useful; a mother recently told me that she used her knuckle ('knuckling in') with a good deal of force and kneaded the clog out. Then she fed on that side until the baby emptied that breast. One of the best tips I've come across is from my lactation consultant friend Mia who suggests using an electric toothbrush on the affected area of a plugged duct, which often breaks up the plugs.

Another suggestion (although no conclusive studies) to help unplug a duct or avoid one completely is to increase your intake of lecithin to **550mg per day**. Lecithin is basically a fat derived from choline and is found in eggs, cheese, yogurt, milk, soy, legumes (fruit or veg grown in a pod like peas), fish, seafood, Brussel sprouts and broccoli. One egg has 147 mg of choline. Other foods high in choline include shrimp (4 oz. = 154 mg), scallops (4 oz. = 126 mg) and swiss chard (1 cup – 50 mg). Lecithin is also sold as a supplement in pharmacies and health food stores and you often see it as an additive in foods.

Occasionally a woman develops a milk *bleb* (blister) on her nipple. A bleb is a blockage of the nipple pore where milk gets trapped under the skin and is more common in women who have a plugged duct. There are several ways of healing it including piercing it with a sterile needle, soaking it with an Epsom salt solution followed by a hot wet compress or a using a heavy duty pump after applying heat. Do your homework on treating a bleb if you develop one and see your healthcare provider if you are unsuccessful in getting rid of it.

If bacteria from the surface of the breast or baby's mouth gets into clogged milk, an infection called **mastitis** can result. Watch for fever, chills, tiredness and/or a large red patch on the breast. A case of mastitis can overtake you and result in a hospital stay if not treated quickly. A recent Doctor in my class told me to tell women "not to wait until you have a fever of 105 °F!" Contact your care provider if you believe that the clogged duct has got worse. Usually you would be prescribed anti-biotics to kill off the bacteria after an examination.

UNDERSTAND JAUNDICE'S UNDERLYING CAUSE

Assuming you can breastfeed and colostrum is present after the baby is born, the first problem mothers and babies often run into is **jaundice**. This is a common condition in newborns with degrees of severity. In actual fact, jaundice is one of nature's protective antioxidants most of the time. **Severe jaundice in the first 24 hours** of birth is _unusual_ and can result in some horrible conditions including brain damage and should be treated immediately.

However most all babies will show signs of jaundice (**skin turning a shade of yellow as bilirubin levels increase** and the baby's immature liver struggles to cope) on day 3-4. This is referred to as **physiologic jaundice**. The underlying problem of physiologic jaundice at day 3-4 is that the baby is probably **not _swallowing_ enough breastmilk** (even though he/she may be nursing a lot)! Let me repeat that: _the baby is not swallowing enough breastmilk_. In addition to phototherapy light treatment ('bili lights'), it is important that you get more milk into the baby any which way you can.

Consider changing positions or get help latching deeper. I'll never forget my midwife's words when my baby turned yellow on day three: "Feed, feed, feed the baby" to clear the jaundice. If breastfeeding isn't working well enough, **feeding some expressed milk, banked milk or formula (using a supplemental nursing system if necessary - pg. 158)** are all helpful solutions. It can be daunting and difficult to express or pump on Day 3 so expressing and storing some colostrum at 38+ weeks for just such an occasion can be a very useful ounce to have on hand in the freezer.

POTENTIAL NEWBORN STOMACH PROBLEMS

We often make assumptions about the root cause of a baby's gassiness, crying or spitting up. From the following chart, you can see how similar many of the esophageal, stomach and small intestine symptoms can be and how difficult it is to pinpoint exactly what is causing the baby's problem.

STOMACH & SMALL INTESTINE PROBLEMS

WHAT'S WRONG?	Spitting-up Reflux or Vomiting	Pain/Crying	Gassiness
GER/GERD	☐☐☐	☐☐	
Colic	☐	☐☐	☐☐
Pyloric Stenosis	☐☐☐ (often & projectile)	☐	
Foremilk Oversupply		☐	☐☐ (green foamy stools)
Galactosemia	☐		☐ (diarrhea)
Formula proteins immune response		☐☐	☐☐
Immune response (allergy) to something in mother's diet/breastmilk		☐☐	☐☐ (loose stool, mucus & blood)

☐ - often
☐☐ - considerable
☐☐☐ - always

IS IT REALLY COLIC?

Colic is a word that is more of a general condition rather than a pin-pointed problem. *It is defined as three or more hours a day of crying for three or more days a week for at least three weeks.* Generally colic starts around the 2-4 week mark and ends somewhere around the 3-4 month mark. Symptoms include the baby being **inconsolable** after a feed (breast or bottle), crying, **getting worse as the day wears on (especially at night),** the baby pulling up or straightening his/her legs and the passing of **gas.**

There are many theories surrounding the cause of **colic** – some thought to center on the mother's diet; others on the immature gut lining – and currently there is no cure. There is a theory that the baby may be receiving too much (of the harder to digest) foremilk and not enough hindmilk. **Some mothers find that adding probiotics to their own diet can greatly help the baby's colic**. Helping the baby to relieve gas (by 'bicycling' the baby's legs) is also welcome. Often rocking the baby or wearing them in a sling helps most of all. Talk to your Pediatrician for a diagnosis and suggestions for helping the baby and see if you can rule out other things (see chart pg. 143).

Gastro Esophageal Reflux (GER) is caused by milk backing up in the baby's esophagus. It causes the baby to spit up after most feeds although it usually looks worse than it is and many babies spit up at some point after a feed. If the baby is spitting up a considerable amount and not gaining weight, you should contact your care provider. **Gastro Esophageal Reflux Disease (GERD)** is a more severe form of GER and is different in that it may involve projectile vomiting and pain.

Babies with GERD are particularly uncomfortable lying down and may arch their back – probably due to pain from heartburn. The baby may also pull away from the breast during a feed or refuse to eat. Try feeding the baby in as upright a position as possible (like the frontal or semi-reclining position). Both GERD and GER usually resolve themselves without treatment but both can be very frustrating, messy and worrying for the parent.

A little known condition called **Pyloric Stenosis** (more common in boys) is when the valve between the stomach and the small intestine is skinny and stops or slows down the contents of the stomach from going into the small intestine. Babies with pyloric stenosis often projectile vomit. This condition usually resolves itself but occasionally surgery is necessary.

COULD IT BE LACTOSE INTOLERANCE?

My son once told me he was *black toast intolerant* when I burned his toast! Despite his misunderstanding of the phrase, lactose intolerance is now in the daily vocabulary of the masses and gets blamed for just about everything gastric. Although common in adults, the condition is generally misdiagnosed in babies.

Our bodies create an enzyme called **lactase** which is used to break down milk sugar (also known as lactose). As an aging adult, the body can start to slow down its ability to produce lactase causing a number of symptoms (including gassiness, diarrhea, bloating and pain) after eating or drinking milk/dairy (lactose). Babies who are premature are often temporarily lactose intolerant until their bodies begin producing lactase. Otherwise this *slowdown* in lactase creation **is almost non-existent** in newborns.

For the tiny percentage of babies that are born truly lactose intolerant, it is probably **inherited (congenital)** and is apparent in the *first few days* of life. Interestingly, it is not a lifelong condition – usually resolving itself in the first six months. However after birth, lactose intolerance can be caused by **damage to the baby's sensitive gut lining**. This can be caused by an **allergy (immune response) from**

an ingredient in formula or a component of breastmilk from the mother's diet.

A specific allergen is often hard to diagnose because it can be virtually impossible to figure out exactly what food or preservative is causing the response. Babies can develop **a milk protein (casein and whey) allergy** to the dairy in their mother's own diet. Processed foods can have lots of additives that *could* be causing the problem. It is useful to keep a food diary listing what you have eaten and the baby's symptoms that follow. It can be real detective work to figure out the culprit. Removing the allergen from breastmilk can normally allow the gut to heal and the intolerance to fade fairly quickly.

WHAT ELSE COULD IT BE?

Many other infant conditions cause gassiness and pain. The first possibility is ***Lactose Overload/Foremilk Oversupply***. When a baby is moved from one breast to another after only a few minutes, 'snacks' or does not latch deeply, he/she may be getting milk with less fat compared to milk higher up in the ducts. Although the terms foremilk and hindmilk are no longer used, the principle is the same: the longer the baby is on the same breast, the better the chances of getting higher fat milk. Milk fat helps to balance the gut and tame gassiness. Too much lactose and not enough fat can cause *green, watery or foamy diapers* and general stomach pain. Keep the baby on the first breast as long as possible (10+ minutes of active sucking as a guide). If you have a 'snacker', you may consider pumping first so that the baby is more likely to receive higher fat milk when breastfeeding.

The second possibility (for babies supplemented with artificial breast milk/formula) is that ***formula is often harder to digest*** than breast milk proteins because of the size of the protein molecules and the occasional immune response inducing reaction. The double whammy effect can cause gassiness and pain after a feed. Realizing the problem, formula manufacturers offer formula that is easier to digest because it has gone through the process of **hydrolysis**. *If your baby needs supplementation with formula and is less than one month old, consider buying partially hydrolyzed ready-made formula for several weeks.*

The third possibility (with symptoms like diarrhea, vomiting and jaundice in the first few days of life) is called **_Galactosemia_**. This is a **_rare condition_** (1 in 30,000 – 60,000 babies and more common in babies of Irish descent) where the baby's body cannot manufacture the liver enzyme GALT. If you can't produce Galt, you can't breakdown lactose either. Babies with true galactosemia should be weaned to soy based milk quickly and may never be able to process lactose without the potential for harm.

AVOID NIPPLE PREFERENCE

When a baby takes milk from a bottle, the flow is often faster and uses far less energy than from a breast. You can see this first hand if you hold a bottle of milk upside down and watch it start to drip. For years, we have been holding the baby flat in our arms and positioning a bottle at an angle so that a relative avalanche of milk comes down into the baby's mouth without much effort. Is it any wonder that babies start to prefer the instant gratification of a bottle over the harder work of pulling it out of the breast?

Putting the breast in a baby's mouth after a bottle feeding could confuse them. This so-called **_nipple confusion_** or more accurately **_nipple preference_** can become a real problem if the baby starts to refuse to be breastfed. In order to avoid this drama, it is suggested that you wait until the four week mark when breastfeeding is well established to introduce anything other than a real nipple (no silicone nipples or pacifiers/dummies). BUT if you are supplementing for medical reason, do not worry about the baby developing nipple preference; **just feed the baby**.

If you are bottle feeding because you are supplementing, exclusively pumping or mixing, you can use *pace feeding* to create a feed that is much more similar to breastfeeding. First sit the baby almost upright (as opposed to horizontal in the crook of your arm) and stroke the silicone teat on the baby's lips like you would if breastfeeding.

When the baby lunges, keep the bottle at a flat 180 degree angle so that the flow is much slower than when the bottle is at a steeper angle. Finally, slow or pause the baby's feed by pulling the milk back into the bottle occasionally. This technique can also help reduce overfeeding. Don't worry about air bubbles when pace feeding. The baby will quickly learn to regulate his or her breathing when feeding to keep the swallowing of air bubbles to a minimum.

RECOGNIZE REVERSE CYCLING

Occasionally clever babies 'reverse cycle' when given formula or breast milk from a bottle. Reverse cycling is the term for *taking just enough milk from a bottle to stave off hunger*. Babies do this because they prefer the breast – a kind of natural addiction to being fed by his/her mother skin to skin where the baby can see or smell her. If the mother is around, they will possibly fuss until the breast is offered. Have someone other than the mother – with all her good smelling breastmilk – give the baby the bottle. You can't really blame them!

IS THE BABY ON A NURSING STRIKE?

The polar opposite of reverse cycling is a **nursing strike**. Imagine the baby happily breastfeeding and then one day pulling away, refusing to latch, crying and fussing at feeding time. Nursing strikes can occur at any time but are usually caused by a baby trying to tell you something. Perhaps the baby is in pain (from new teeth, a healing lip or tongue tie snip, gas when put in a certain position), ill (can't breathe if nose is stuffed up when feeding), stressed (you reacted loudly last time the baby fed because he accidentally bit you or you've been away for a long time), distracted (because the baby has been overstimulated with many visitors) or reacting to a slow let down (compared to the instant gratification of the bottle). Another motive for strike can be taste: sometimes milk tastes different to the baby depending on what the mother is eating or if she becomes pregnant again.

Nursing strikes can be very upsetting for the mother who is only ever trying to do her best. Figuring out the root of the problem is like being a detective. Keep trying and keep the baby skin to skin as much as you can for a few days. Check the baby's gums for signs of teeth. Think about what you are eating and any recent changes to diet or lifestyle. If the baby just won't nurse, you can pump if possible. Usually the baby will eventually return to the breast.

NOBODY TOLD ME ABOUT THRUSH!

A friend of mine who I went to visit a week after her daughter's birth stated those exact words loudly to me at her front door so I'm forewarning you to be on the lookout for this fungal infection! Thrush is caused by the **overgrowth** of a fungus which every baby has in his/her mouth. It is usually easy to spot because of the characteristic **white blotches on the baby's tongue or gums**.

One of the first symptoms (besides the white blotched tongue) is a **fussy, cranky baby** at feeding times due to pain. The mother often gets **itchy nipples** which may also turn red, crack and become highly sensitive. Sometimes her areola becomes a bit shiny or itchy too. Finally, some women with thrush experience deep, **stabbing pains** when they are breastfeeding or painful nipples when not feeding. It is easy for the baby to pass the infection to his/her mother and vice versa so recognizing it and getting treated quickly by your doctor is important.

DOES LET DOWN BRING YOU WAY DOWN?

The final problem in this chapter is the relatively recent realization that when some women let-down (signal to the brain to turn on the milk ejection reflex at the beginning of a feed), they experience negative feelings ranging from mild self-correcting symptoms (homesickness, hopelessness, depression) often lasting less than three months to moderate ones (panic, agitation, paranoia) that may carry on for 6-12 months or longer. This 30 seconds (or more) of misery is a condition referred to as **D-MER (Dysphoric Milk Ejection Reflex)** and is thought to be connected to rapidly dropping dopamine levels when the mother lets down.

While it is becoming easier to spot a woman suffering from D-MER, possible solutions are not as easy to identify. Some women are prescribed the dopamine reuptake inhibitor Bupropion while others turn to the Siberian herb Rhodiola (Arctic Root) in capsule form. Just recognizing the condition seems the first step in helping women deal with the emotional aspect of the syndrome. Finally, a few online resources and social support groups have sprung up including www.D-MER.org and the Facebook support group associated with the website.

PHONE A FRIEND OR MAKE AN APPOINTMENT

My niece told me that the hardest part of breastfeeding for her was at 3.30am when the baby wouldn't latch, she was in tears and her partner just wanted to sleep! As I've said before, breastfeeding is both an art and a science. Overcoming problems depends on many factors and support is often the difference between carrying on and quitting. The key is surrounding yourself with a supportive tribe of people who can help you if times get tough.

Contacting your friend who jacked in breastfeeding on day 3 to talk about latching issues is about as useful as getting driving advice from someone who has never been behind the wheel. Before you go into labor, line up a few friends, relatives or acquaintances that have breastfed successfully and put their contact details in your phone! She may be able to loan you a pump, talk you off the formula cliff, recommend a possible solution or spot something you hadn't noticed. At the very least, she can make you a cup of tea and remind you that you are doing a great job.

Also, consider attending support groups with like-minded parents. One of the only reasons that I remained sane during the first three months of having a new baby was the weekly coffee mornings I attended with women on my street. We started off as complete strangers but having a new baby in common gives you a lot to talk about for the next 18 years. Many birth centers, hospitals and clinics also offer breastfeeding circles or support groups. The lactation support group I run dries the tears of those women with problems very quickly. It is good to have others listen, relate and give suggestions.

Finally, seek out a ***lactation specialist*** (IBC Lactation Consultant) to diagnose and correct problems when you cannot. While most work in the hospital or clinic setting, some do private work and even make house calls. Getting help early is one of the best ways to sort out a problem before its roots take hold.

SUMMARY

☐ Women who have hormonal imbalances, had breast surgery or breast development issues may struggle with milk production or latching. Plan on breastfeeding and speak to your care provider in advance to understand where and when to get help locally if problems do arise.

☐ Physiologic jaundice at day 3-4 is common and the underlying problem is that the baby is not **swallowing** enough breastmilk.

☐ Colic is a more general term for crying and digestion issues. Many conditions have overlapping symptoms and it can be difficult to pinpoint the underlying cause. Most conditions resolve themselves eventually without treatment.

☐ True lactose intolerance in babies is exceptionally rare. However adult-like symptoms of lactose intolerance in babies are more likely to be caused by an allergy to something in the mother's diet, foremilk overload, galactosemia or the struggle to digest larger formula milk protein molecules.

☐ Blocked ducts can lead to mastitis. Clear a blocked duct with warmth, cold, massage and breastfeeding. If a mastitis infection sets in, see your care provider for treatment.

☐ Pace feeding mimics breastfeeding and can help a baby overcome nipple preference or confusion.

☐ Reverse cycling is when a baby takes only enough milk from a bottle to satisfy hunger pangs instead of feeling full. These babies prefer breastfeeding.

☐ Nursing strikes usually occur when the baby is trying to tell you something.

☐ Thrush is a common overgrowth of a fungus that lives in the baby's mouth. It is easy to identify because of the white blotches on the baby's tongue. The mother's symptoms include itchiness or shiny skin on the areola and deep stabbing pain in the breast. Getting treated quickly is important.

☐ Feeling negative emotions when you let down is a recognized condition abbreviated D-MER. Symptoms vary but arctic root capsules may help. Alternatively, contact your care provider for help (and tell them about Dysphoric Milk Ejection Reflex because they may have never heard of it).

☐ Think ahead and make contact with a woman who can help support you if a breastfeeding problem arises. Spend a few minutes researching local support groups, breastfeeding circles and lactation consultants. Don't be afraid to ask questions or get help.

FINDING THE CULPRIT – KAREN'S STORY

My sweet baby Johannah was born a month premature after I was induced due to my leaking bag of water. Despite the early arrival, she was healthy at 5 lbs. 8 oz. I had planned on breastfeeding her and she latched beautifully. I was smitten by both her and breastfeeding.

We did struggle to wake her for feeds. She was a sleepy eater and it was difficult to arouse her. My husband gently flicked her feet if my methods didn't work. She also returned to the hospital for two days in the NICU under the bili lights to help clear her jaundice. We brought home a small but otherwise healthy little girl.

We were home for about a month or so when the symptoms of colic kicked in. From about 7-10pm every night, she would wail! During these sessions, she was gassy and uncomfortable and the only soothing techniques that helped were movement and 'shushing' (two of the 5 calming techniques made famous by Dr Harvey Karp). Next her bowel movements started loosening to the point of liquid. Then the liquid turned to blood and mucus and I knew we had a bigger problem than colic.

Luckily my husband is a pediatrician and sees symptoms like this when babies develop an allergy to something their mother is eating and passing through to them via breastmilk. We managed to collect a stool sample from her for testing. Viral and bacterial infections were ruled out. Milk protein was the suspected culprit.

In order to prove the milk protein allergy, I had to choose between dropping all milk proteins (called casein and whey) from my own diet or move her to a soy based formula. I decided that there wasn't anything I wouldn't do for my gorgeous little girl and so I gave up dairy. I had no idea how hard it would be. Casein and whey are found in every milk product derived from a mammal. No ice cream, yogurt, milk or butter allowed. I also had to eliminate bread, crackers and thousands of other products where casein and whey are used as additives or thickeners. I had to be SO diligent. I even found some 'vegan' cheese that contained casein and whey! The worst part was pouring my precious store of frozen pumped milk down the drain and starting over.

For the next 10 months of breastfeeding, I watched everything I ate. Removing dairy from my diet made me *skinny and mean*! I remember going to an Italian restaurant where there was nothing on the menu that I could eat except plain noodles with olive oil. Reading labels became a big part of my life. Johannah's recovery was not instantaneous – it took about five weeks for her symptoms to completely clear – including the nightly crying. After she healed, life was so much easier.

She never grew out of the allergy. I became the 'snack mom' who made dairy free cupcakes on her birthday. If she ever has a stomach issue, I immediately become the food detective by examining the ingredients in her diet. Often new symptoms are a result of the manufacturer changing the ingredients in a 'safe' favorite - usually the addition of a milk protein. Johannah still has a sensitive stomach and has eliminated dairy (and later eggs). If she accidentally eats something she shouldn't, her body reacts quickly.

Looking back on the experience, I was lucky that my husband diagnosed her so fast. I probably would have just put up with my 'colicky' baby and not realized that the symptoms of colic often have a more serious underlying cause. Since no one else in my family has a food allergy, we certainly weren't expecting one. I don't think that we, as humans, are meant to have mammal's milk forever anyway.

AUTHOR'S NOTE: Karen's food detective skills have taught me a great deal about food allergens. She continues to be an exemplary mom, educator and friend!

CHAPTER 11

FEEDING THE PREMATURE OR SPECIAL NEEDS BABY

__BREASTFEEDING DOESN'T HAVE TO SUCK__ if you work with the needs of the baby for the best possible outcome.

Babies with special needs benefit immensely from breastmilk. The issue is often getting the milk into them. Breastfeeding the special needs baby doesn't have to suck if you work out the logistics of balancing the baby's health needs with a breastfeeding and/or pumping plan.

FEED THE PREMATURE BABY ANY WAY YOU CAN

Babies born before term (38 weeks) or small (less than 5 lbs.) are often smaller, sleepier babies and that can make feeding them a lot harder. They are often not able to latch well (or at all) and will need feeding at regular intervals. Most hospitals have premium hospital grade breast pumps for the mothers to use while the baby is in the neonatal intensive care unit (NICU) and often for the first 30-60 days after the baby is brought home. Many mothers find hand expressing –

especially in the early days – more efficient than an electric pump when they get the hang of it.

Cup feeding is one way to get pumped milk into a tiny mouth. It helps to stimulate the baby's instinct to suck. With the milk right by their lip, they take small amounts slowly and are able to control the pace at which they transfer and swallow. Cup feeding is also used for older babies who are refusing a bottle after being exclusively breast fed. Most any small cup can be used including plastic medicine measuring cups or specifically designed Nifty cups®. Cup feeding takes some practice getting the tilt of the cup right so that the baby laps, sips or slurps the milk instead of a gag inducing pour. Usually 15-20 minutes (with a burp half way through) of feeding is adequate without over-tiring the baby.

Another feeding technique for small sleepy babies is called *Finger Feeding*. This method is closer to breastfeeding than cup feeding and can help coordinate the suck reflex for future breastfeeding. Using the index finger (pad upward, nail downward) and the feeding tube of the supplemental nursing system (SNS) attached to a milk source, the parent inserts both into the baby's mouth to mimic the breast. As the baby sucks both the finger and the tube together, the milk is drawn into the baby's mouth. If your baby is in the NICU, the staff will assist you. Otherwise a lactation consultant can also coach you through finger feeding.

The *least popular but potentially most rewarding* method of establishing a latch with a premature, small or sleepy baby is using the **supplemental nursing system (SNS)** at the breast instead of using a finger. The mother puts the nipple and as much of her areola as the baby can manage into the baby's mouth along with the feeding tube. This mimics breastfeeding more than any other method because the baby must create a vacuum with the breast to receive milk. It is also used in the early days (day 2-10+) if the mother's milk is slow to dilute and increase in volume and allows for skin to skin bonding.

CLEFT LIP AND PALATE

Both the baby's lips and roof of the mouth (palate) develop in the first trimester of pregnancy. For unknown reasons, sometimes the baby's body tissue does not join together completely causing a division or split (*cleft*) on the lip and/or roof of the mouth (palate). The incidence is estimated to be roughly1 in every 690 births.

A small cleft on the roof of the mouth may not be noticed or need treatment. A baby that spits up or vomits through his or her nose probably has a soft palate cleft. A cleft on the lip can also go up into the nose. Surgery is normally performed in the first few months to correct both the appearance and functionality of the baby's nose and mouth and the baby is normally attended by a cleft palate/craniofacial team.

Most babies with a cleft palate have feeding challenges because they cannot make an efficient mouth seal on the breast. The mother would be issued a hospital grade pump and can feed the baby pumped breastmilk using a bottle specifically designed for babies with a cleft. She can also allow the baby to suckle the breast to bond and benefit from skin to skin contact even though it may be non-nutritive (not specifically for a feed). The American Cleft Palate-Craniofacial Association (**www.acpa-cpf.org**) has a wealth of information on their website including feeding instructions in the *Feeding Your Baby* video series.

HEART DEFECTS

A baby with a heart defect (a hole in the wall, a connection between blood vessels that narrows, fails to close, stays open, a blockage, reduced blood flow, etc.) will benefit greatly from breastmilk but may (or may not) also require additional caloric supplementation. Often care providers are hesitant to promote breastfeeding because of the worry that the extra energy required to do so will put a strain on the existing condition.

However research tells us that breastfed babies have higher levels of oxygen saturation and blood flow while feeding. They may also gain weight faster than a formula-fed infant with the same defect leading to a faster release from hospital. Finally the immunities passed through to the baby from the mother will assist the baby in fighting off infection.

Parents should be aware that the defect may cause the baby to feed slower and require more breaks. Supplementing with pumped hindmilk after a feed and using a SNS can be particularly effective. The *supine, semi-reclining or football hold* (pgs. 87-91) positions can also help reduce fatigue while feeding.

OTHER SPECIAL NEEDS

Babies who are born with *spina bifida* and other neural tube defects usually benefit greatly from skin to skin contact and breastfeeding. Most babies diagnosed with spina bifida are delivered via C-Section and moved to the NICU immediately so hand expressing colostrum may be necessary in the first three days. Mothers will usually be issued a hospital grade pump. C-Sections can separate the mother and baby for those first few hours so reconnect skin to skin as soon as possible.

Babies are screened for *blood disorders (such as sickle cell disease and thalassemia)* after they are born and roughly 307,000 babies are diagnosed globally per year. There are rare situations in which the baby is in a poor condition at birth and cannot latch but most babies will happily breastfeed.

Downs Syndrome (Trisomy 21) affects over 217,000 babies born every year worldwide. These babies can have trouble with latching on to the breast due to low muscle tone. They can also have problems swallowing. Similar to premature babies however, breastmilk is important to their health going forward.

Roughly 177,000 babies are born annually with *Glucose-6-Phosphate Dehydrogenase (G6PD)*. This is a metabolic disorder where the baby's blood breaks down during oxidative stress (caused by eating or ingesting certain foods or drugs). This can impair the baby's liver causing bilirubin problems. The condition can be mild or severe. Breastfeeding is believed to be the best way forward but the mother's diet (and breastmilk components) can affect the condition. Mothers should avoid eating *fava (broad) beans* (this disorder was originally called favism due to fava bean triggers) or using henna (skin or hair products) as well as several anti-biotics (check with your care provider).

SUMMARY:

☐ Feeding a *premature baby, small baby or special needs baby* can be a challenge. Cup feeding stimulates the baby's instinct to suck. Finger feeding can be useful with a sleepy baby. A supplemental nursing system (SNS) most closely mimics breastfeeding because the baby must create a vacuum to draw milk. However once the baby grows bigger and stronger, breastfeeding is a great comfort to both the mother and baby.

☐ Feeding a baby with a cleft lip and/or palate can be a challenge. Babies with this issue usually respond well to pumped breastmilk in a special bottle. Also allowing the baby to suckle at the breast is beneficial for bonding and all the benefits of skin to skin contact.

☐ Babies with heart defects may tire more easily when breastfeeding and require more breaks. Feeding in upright positions and combining breastfeeding with a SNS is a useful combination.

☐Breastmilk is beneficial to all babies with special needs. Breastfeeding may or may not be possible but care providers should be able to give specialist help if needed.

THE PATH LESS TRAVELLED – SUZANNE'S STORY

Ryan was born nine days past his due date - induced after my water broke. He was a healthy weight at 7lb 6oz but I knew immediately that something wasn't right. The staff was very quiet. Ryan didn't cry right away and had low Apgar scores. After letting me see him for a minute, he was whisked away to the NICU and that is where he remained for the next twelve days.

While I was recovering from labor, I found out that Ryan had a seizure in the NICU. As soon as I could manage, I went down to see him. I watched a merry-go-round of doctors come in to observe and treat him. At some point he was given antibiotics which I believe may have caused problems later on in his gut development. Eventually he was diagnosed with polycythemia (extra red blood cells which can block the flow of blood), a heart defect and a few other problems. Slowly however, he began to improve.

Once I was discharged, I went back and forth to the hospital every four hours. In the first few days Ryan was too weak to latch so I pumped the best I could. My daily routine became early morning pumping, going to the hospital to feed him, coming home to soak in the tub to help relax, pumping again and then going back to the hospital.

By day 5, my milk was abundant and I was able to pump and store milk at home but also breastfeed him in the hospital. He was a bit of a sleepy eater but he latched well. We brought Ryan home on Day 13. The next few months and years would be a voyage of discovery about his health but I managed to breastfed him for 16 months. I felt it was the best thing I could do for him. It was around the end of my breastfeeding relationship with Ryan that I found out I was pregnant again.

In the fourth month of my second pregnancy, I found out that our baby had a triple copy of chromosome 21 – also known as Downs Syndrome. My husband and I were both accepting of this diagnosis and carried on with the pregnancy. A month before the baby was due, I was told to go in for weekly non-stress tests (NSTs). Three days after my first NST, I got a call telling me to come in for induction because I had low amniotic fluid.

Although I feared the worst, Ethan was born incredibly healthy. He weighted 6lb 13 oz. with Apgar scores of 9. He was beautiful. He had none of the heart defects nor low muscle tone that can plague Downs' babies. The only challenge with Ethan was feeding. Not only did he not latch on to the breast, he didn't seem interested in eating at all. I started pumping after we discovered that he would feed happily from a bottle. Just like with the early days of Ryan, pumping became part of the daily regime. However after four months of pumping, we moved over to formula. With a special needs toddler running around, I felt overwhelmed and exhausted. It was definitely the right move for us.

I feel so incredibly lucky to have my two boys. Years later I found out that a nurse had said something very negative to my husband about carrying on with a Downs Syndrome pregnancy. I still think about that nurse and how wrong she was. My advice to new parents – especially those of children with special needs – is to use any support that is offered. My family, friends and community all pitched in and that is how we survived. Sometimes it really does take a village.

AUTHOR'S NOTE: Suzanne's story continues to be a journey. Today her boys are thriving although they still have regular doctor's appointments for conditions associated with their births. They are an amazing family and she is an amazing mother.

CHAPTER 12

LEARN ABOUT PUMPING, CATCHING & STORING MILK

BREASTFEEDING DOESN'T HAVE TO SUCK if you feel knowledgeable and confident using a variety of breast pumps and equipment.

As mentioned in Chapter 9, many women give up breastfeeding at the three day or two week mark because they just don't think they have enough milk or because the baby is struggling to latch deeply causing pain. This chapter outlines the many ways to feed a baby breastmilk from a bottle by pumping or catching milk.

LEARN TO HAND EXPRESS EARLY

One of the oldest global techniques for increasing milk supply is to *hand express* a bit of milk before or after a feed. Expressing makes you appreciate every single drop you produce because it can seem slow and time consuming at first. Still, it can be done anywhere and without electricity. And, as mentioned previously, it can also greatly increase your supply if done in the early days after birth.

IN ORDER TO HAND EXPRESS:

1. First gently massage the breast in a semi-circle about an inch or two above the areola with your finger-tips.
2. Next, cup your thumb and index finger about an inch behind the areola.
3. The third step is to gently push in about half an inch towards your body and then gently squeeze your cupped hand together. Then repeat. Think to yourself: *PRESS, COMPRESS, RELAX, REPEAT.*

Hand express in a rhythmic fashion and alternate to the other breast after every ten or so compressions. **It can take at least a minute or two for your body to let down.** You can catch the drops you produce with a teaspoon, cup, bowl, bottle or sterile container.

An inexpensive **manual hand pump** is sometimes easier than hand expressing because it creates suction which stimulates let down. There are many brands on the market which all do the same thing. Considerations include the price, comfort level, suction strength, bottle attachments and how many hands are required.

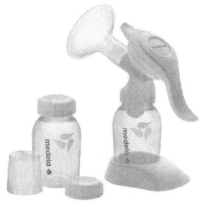

Medela ® manual hand pump

If hand expressing or hand pumping is too daunting, try the **'warm jar' method**. This involves filling a 2.5 in/6 cm wide jar with (very) warm water, then draining it and letting the rim cool so you don't burn yourself. Next center the jar over the nipple and hold against the skin. A vacuum forms as the jar cools and draws milk from the breast! It is an old but effective method.

CATCH MILK ANOTHER WAY!

One of the newest manual hand pumps on the market today is not a pump at all but rather a *milk catcher* like the warm jar. The Haakaa® (pg. 126), Baby Anigo® and Zenda® are a few of the many brand names of **passive pumps** that are used only when you are breastfeeding. With the baby feeding on one breast, the passive pump is suctioned on to the other and catches any drops that you let down.

Many women report collecting over an ounce or more of milk with a passive pump attached. Many of these *catchers* come with a lid allowing you to put the container directly in the fridge in case it is needed during the *'witching hours'* (from 5-7pm) when most women's bodies are at their lowest energy level and babies are at their most tired or fussy.

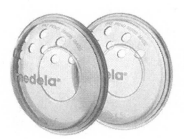

Another milk catcher (and also nipple protector and nipple eversion trainer) is called a **breast shell (pictured)**. The shell is worn inside the bra between feeds and protects the nipple from touching clothing or being irritated against a wet breast pad. It also has the added benefit of collecting any drops of milk that may leak out in between feeds.

Women report everted nipples staying more prominent when wearing breast shells. One downside to be aware of is that when you lean forward, milk that has collected in the shell may spill out through the air holes. It only takes a few mishaps before you learn to squat straight down instead of leaning over when wearing a shell.

PUMP IT UP BY MACHINE

Choosing and using an electric pump can be a stressful and daunting experience. With so many pumps on the market, how do you choose? Pumps are like cars: they basically all do the same thing. Cars get you from one place to another and pumps move milk from the breast to a container. It is the speed, power, style and comfort that varies between models and makes some far more expensive than others.

Consumer pumps also vary in whether they offer battery use (for on the go), hands-free pumping, a let down setting, etc. Some are more efficient, some fit better, others make less noise and many allow you to walk around without being attached to a machine (Freemie®, Willow®, Elvie®). The best idea is to ask friends for recommendations, read reviews and then make a decision – just like buying a car. The website **www.legendairymilk.com** and Instagram blog has zillions of pump/ing tips. Many health insurers cover the cost of a pump up to a certain dollar amount.

For parents who have a baby in the Neo Natal Intensive Care Unit (NICU), hospital grade pumps are usually made available for use by the mother. Hospital pumps equate to the Mercedes Benz of cars and include brands like Medela Symphony ®, Ameda Elite ® and Ardo Medical Carum ®. They normally cost well over $1000+ and are often not sold in retail stores. Occasionally you can rent one or buy one second-hand.

Electric pumps can also be quite daunting for the sleep-deprived, stressed-out mother to put together. Besides the actual pump, you will probably also receive a power adapter (check to see if your pump will automatically switch from battery to electricity if batteries are in), tubing, connectors, valves, membranes, bottles (containers) and flanges (also called breast shields or horns). It may be easiest to start assembling from the flange and work your way towards the machine.

Putting a pump on the breast should be straightforward but occasionally the flange needs to be swapped out for a smaller or larger size. The standard size flange (24-27mm) is thought to be the diameter of the average nipple. When centering the flange on the breast, the nipple should be able to move freely and should not be touching the sides. The areola should not be drawn into the breast pump tunnel. Finally, the pump should not cause you any damage or pain! A good fit should allow a comfortable experience with good results.

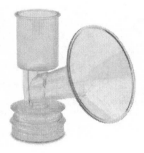

Breast Pump Flanges come in different sizes

Earlier I mentioned a let down setting on some pumps. If your pump does not have a let down setting, start by having the speed high (100%) but the suction lower (70%) to mimic the baby's fast sucking that stimulates let down. After milk starts dropping, turn the pump speed down (30%) but increase the suction (95%) in order to mimic the baby's natural rhythm of slower but deeper sucking. Be gentle on yourself and find your comfort level. Pumping shouldn't hurt.

Remember that pumping is triggered by oxytocin release and many women struggle to pump when stressed or tired. Consider **covering up when you pump** or putting a sock over the bottle so you don't get disheartened when the bottle isn't filling as fast as you'd like.

Perhaps the best pumping tip has to do with the angle at which the flange (horn or breast shield) attaches to the breast. The most obvious position to have the attachment is straight out in front of you so milk drips directly down into the bottle. For whatever reason, turning the *bottle* about 20 degrees either direction on the breast causes less, if any, leakage! Finally, be on the lookout for a kink in your tubing which could cause a loss of suction or power.

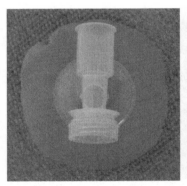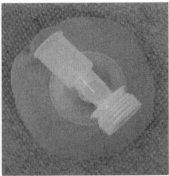

HANDS ON COMBO PUMP FOR MORE MILK!

Using an electric pump is a popular way to remove milk from the breast but it is believed that most electric pumps only remove 50% of the available milk. In a 2009 study by Dr Jane Morton (Journal of Perinatology), women were able to remove 100% more milk from the breast if they used an electric pump **while massaging and compressing the upper breast at the same time**. This is referred to as Combination (Combo) or *Hands On Pumping (HOP)*.

To see a useful demonstration of women massaging and compressing the larger part of their breast while the pump works the lower half, watch 'Maximizing Milk Production' on the **www.med.stanford.edu** website. In addition to Hands On Pumping, women in the same study also found that they could **hand express additional milk out of the breast after the pump no longer worked**! It would seem that pumps are useful for removing the milk closest to the surface but both combo pumping and expressing after the pump no longer draws any out is even more effective.

UNDERSTAND CHANGING MILK COLOR

When pumping, women are often alarmed by the varying color of milk they produce! Changing milk color is very rarely a worry. Remember that colostrum is **golden or orange** and changes to a lighter whiter color in the first week after birth. Occasionally milk may turn back to that darker golden color – often the result of antibodies manufactured by the mother's body for the baby's needs. Also, certain foods eaten by the mother can cause the breastmilk to change other tinges of color. As a general rule of thumb, any food that could stain your clothing or turn your tongue a certain color could also alter the appearance of your breastmilk temporarily.

The beta-carotene found in carrots, sweet potatoes and squash may turn milk slightly **yellow or orange**. **Green** colored breastmilk is often the result of eating a lot of green veggies like kale, seaweed or spinach. Green food dyes can also cause green tinted breastmilk. Finally, some *medications* or multi-vitamins (iron) can turn breastmilk **green** (or **black**!).

Occasionally women notice a **pink** tint to breastmilk. This could be caused by naturally red foods (beets or pomegranates) or artificially colored ones. The red tint could also be due to a tiny bit of blood in the milk (from a cracked nipple or broken capillary). Neither red foods nor a temporary pink tinge are normally an ongoing concern but do contact your care provider if in doubt. However if the pink milk leaves a stain on the inside of a bottle, a rare bacteria called *Serratia Marcescens* may be the culprit and needs treatment immediately.

STORAGE TIPS

Milk pumped from your body is not that different from cow's milk in terms of storage. Milk fresh from the body can be left on the counter for roughly four hours in a covered container, stored for 4 days in the coldest part of the fridge (at a constant temp of 40F or colder) or frozen for up to one year. It is best to avoid storing milk containers on the inside of the fridge or freezer door because of the struggle to maintain a constant state of cold due to being opened and shut frequently.

BREAST MILK (Freshly Pumped or Expressed) Storage

WHERE?	HOW LONG?
Room Temp (≤ 77°F/ 25°C)	4 hours
Refrigerator (≤ 40°F/ 4°C)	Up to 4 days
Freezer (≤ 0°F/-18°C)	6 - 12 months

Ref: CDC Human Milk Storage Guidelines 2019

BREAST MILK (Thawed – Previously Frozen) Storage

WHERE?	HOW LONG?
Room Temp (≤ 77°F/ 25°C)	1-2 hours
Refrigerator (≤ 40°F/ 4°C)	Up to 1 day (24 hours)
Freezer (≤ 0°F/-18°C)	NEVER refreeze

Ref: CDC Human Milk Storage Guidelines 2019

When milk sits on the counter or in the fridge, you will usually see it separate into thinner and lighter milk at the top and milk with more fat at the bottom – a bit like raw milk from a cow. When you transfer milk to a freezer bag, leave an inch or so of space at the top because

milk expands when frozen. Also mark on the bag the date, the amount (ounces, ml) and your baby's last name if the baby will be using it at daycare or during travel.

One last tip for the storage of breastmilk it to store breastmilk bags **flat** in the freezer so they freeze level. A clever friend of mine put a small shoe box in her freezer with a ½ inch slit carved out of the front bottom of the box. She stored her milk bags flat in the box and always used the oldest milk first by pulling her milk envelopes through the bottom slot. That way the newer frozen milk was always placed on top in the box and the older milk was used first by pulling it out of the *slot*.

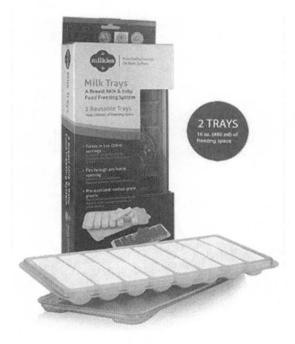

In the last few years a few ice cube trays designed specifically for breastmilk have come on the market and they are usually designed to freeze milk in one ounce bars so that you can decide how many bars you need and unfreeze a more accurate amount. Be aware of any plastic storage containers that have the recycle symbol number 7. This indicates the plastic may contain a common chemical called Bisphenol A (BPA). The US Food and Drug Administration have expressed concern over use and toxicity of plastics containing BPA in humans.

SUMMARY

☐ Hand expressing or using a manual hand pump can be done anywhere and does not rely on electricity. The warm jar method is also effective. Expressing a few drops before and after a feed is one of the best and easiest ways to improve the mother's milk supply long term.

☐ *Milk catchers* are devices which catch milk without actually using a mechanical or electric pump. The passive silicone pump is attached to one breast while you are breastfeeding on the other. Breast shells are attached to the breast and worn inside the bra.

☐ Electric pumps are efficient at removing milk from the breast faster than by hand but combo pumping is the most efficient method. The price of pumps varies but they all do the same basic thing. A good fitting flange (horn, breast shield) is essential.

☐ The ability to pump relies on your ability to relax, let down and let go. Covering up when you pump can make you feel less vulnerable.

☐ Pumped milk can be stored for roughly 4 hours at room temperature, up to a week in a covered container in the coldest part of the fridge and up to a year in the deep freeze. Use the oldest milk in your fridge or freezer first.

CHAPTER 13

PLAN FOR RETURNING TO WORK OR SCHOOL

BREASTFEEDING DOESN'T HAVE TO SUCK if you make a plan ahead of time for when your child will not be with you.

Once the baby is sleeping longer stretches at night and you can count on a stable milk supply, life becomes a lot easier. Looking ahead, you may already be thinking about how you will cope when you go back to work or school. Mothers make caring for a baby look easy although we all realize what a tough but rewarding job it can be. Finding the right person to care for your child and figuring out a feeding and pumping solution is probably one of the most stressful decisions you will face in the first year.

WORK OUT THE LOGISTICS OF CHILDCARE

After I had my first baby, I returned to work after 16 weeks off. Around the 8 week mark, I began investigating nearby nurseries. I had no idea that there might be waiting lists. The first thing you need to work out is who is going to look after your child when you are out of the house and the sooner you can line that up, the better.

I lost many hours of sleep stressing over the cost of childcare and the advantages and disadvantages of a daycare center versus an individual care provider. I also had to take my working hours into consideration to see if I needed help with pickups and drop-offs because many childcare providers have firm hours in which they will (or will not) look after a child with financial penalties for being just a few minutes late.

Then I had to consider how I would cope if my child was sick and couldn't mix with other children at daycare even though I was still paying them AND I had to take off work myself in order to look after my sick child! There are a lot of logistics and decisions to be made and a solution will become apparent for you just like it did for me. Just don't leave it until the last minute.

The next thing to think about is what your child's eating and sleeping habits will be by the time you return to work or school and how many hours you will be away from the baby. Will you be working night shift or days? Will you be able to feed the baby from the breast before you leave for work and when you get home? Or will you need to pump all feeds (except the late night ones)?

At the three month mark, it is likely that the average baby would need about 25 ounces a day spread over six feeds (four or so ounces per feed). If you can feed the baby two of them at home, you would need to pump 3-4 times at work (and approximately 17 ounces in total per day). Will your job allow you the flexibility to pump at regular intervals? Will you be able to let down without your baby in front of you to trigger oxytocin? What will you need to take with you every day for the storage of pumped milk?

FREEZE A WEEKS SUPPLY

One of the questions I'm normally asked is how much milk should be on hand in the freezer or refrigerator for a care provider. In theory, you really only need to have a supply for one day's feeds and perhaps a few extra ounces in case of a growth spurt. In reality however, women often build up a substantial supply of milk that they will probably not need. So somewhere in between a one day supply and a freezer full is probably the *right* answer – perhaps a one week supply is a good goal.

Most pumps come with storage bottles. It is useful to have a fridge/freezer bag to both store (in the work fridge) and haul your daily pumped breastmilk home in. If you freeze milk at work and it thaws on the way home, you should not refreeze it.

PUMP AT THE SAME TIME YOU WOULD HAVE FED

Your body can adjust to pumping 30 minutes later than you did at the same time yesterday but you may find yourself getting a little (or a lot) engorged. Engorgement is uncomfortable and can be embarrassing if you start to leak through clothing. My friend Karen told me that she once hand pumped in the taxi on the way to the airport after a meeting over ran by an hour causing her breasts to engorge. This also messed up her pumping schedule.

As mentioned earlier, you should aim to pump at roughly the same time during the day that your baby would have fed. If possible, schedule meetings, classes and activities around pumping times or vice versa. I've known many women with a hands-free pump kit that pump while driving, however the best place to pump is in a calm environment where you can relax and think about what you are doing and why.

DROP A FEED A WEEK IF GIVING UP COMPLETELY

If you decide to stop pumping or breastfeeding completely, give up slowly. A useful recommendation is to drop one (breast) feed per week while adding one formula feed. If you were breastfeeding five times a day, you should ideally drop breastfeeding over a five week period. It is possible for most women's bodies to manufacture and maintain enough milk for a morning and night feed (pre and post work 10-12 hours apart) but most women notice a dwindling supply.

Eventually the day will come when either you or the child decide it is time to stop. It can be a sad day but often the right time very much presents itself. No matter how long you have breastfed or pumped, any breastfeeding is better than none. Well done for doing it as long as you did! If you want to carry on but your child does not, consider pumping for donor milk banks!

SUMMARY:

☐ Working out the logistics of childcare can be stressful. Investigate your options as soon as possible.

☐ Think in advance about how often your child will need to be fed breastmilk while you are away. Multiply the number of feeds by 4 and that will give you a rough idea of how many ounces you will need to pump and replace on a daily basis.

☐ Make sure you keep pumped milk in the refrigerator or freezer (or in a cold pack) at work or school. Refrigerated milk can be frozen one time only. Once thawed, milk should not be refrozen.

☐ Pump outside of the house at the same time you (or as close as possible) would have breastfed the baby if you had been home.

☐If and when you decide to stop breastfeeding, drop your feeds or pumps slowly (if possible - a feed per week) so you don't engorge and risk a blocked duct or mastitis.

CHRISTEEN'S STORY – GOING BACK TO WORK

I'm a 7th Grade Math Teacher at a California Junior High School and I was able to finish the school year since Lila was born in July. By using a combination of sick days, partial pay and unpaid time I was lucky enough to extend my maternity leave until after the December Holidays when she was nearly six months old.

Before Lila was born, we researched several daycare facilities. We were surprised to find that only a few accepted infants under a year old. The place we liked the most (and eventually chose) had encouraged us to visit other places and take our time selecting the right place for Lila – and that was good advice. Ultimately, we came back to the one that felt most like a family and treated us the same way.

I had always planned on pumping when I returned to work so before I left, a pregnant co-worker and I sat down with our Principal to discuss how it could work with our schedules and where we could pump in private. There was no one spot that was going to be available on campus all day long but the Principal was VERY supportive – even offering his own office at one point! Ultimately, I bought a Freemie® cup and Liberty Pump® that you hook onto your belt loop. The Freemie® cup fits into your bra and allows you to walk around and pump at the same time. The pump is not quite quiet enough to use around the kids but it does allow me to be social at lunch time with other teachers rather than locking myself away alone in a room. As a teacher, I need that social interaction with adults!

Although my work day officially starts at 8am, I start by waking up at 5am and getting myself ready before I get the baby up at 6am to feed and dress her. I leave at 6.30am to drop her at daycare and then get to work for meetings, preparation and occasional yard duty. Pickup time for me is around 3.30pm most days – so eight hours total. I have found that I can make it until lunchtime to pump without getting engorged. When I do (dual) pump, I set the pump's timer for ten minutes. I'm getting between 2 to 4 ounces on each side during a session. I also pump immediately after school finishes. Afterwards, I stash the milk in a mini-fridge, wipe down the pump and parts with disposable wipes and take it all home.

At the daycare, there are a maximum of eight infants (under a year) in the Infant Room with up to four babies per one care provider. That seems like a lot of babies – and sometimes the care provider cannot attend to a crying one while she is feeding another – but overall Lila seems very happy there. Another reason I like the facility we chose is that they use a sophisticated app to send updates (which come through as notifications) all day long instead of a summary paper page at pickup. They also summarize her day (hours napping, diaper counts, etc.) via the app.

Financially, we were prepared for the cost, since we had visited the school before she was born. Our facility charges us a weekly fee and charges us 50% less when she is on vacation. Some daycare centers limit how much vacation you can take but ours does not. The Center was also kind enough to allow Lila to attend only half days during her first week to ease her (and me) into being at daycare and were willing to discuss a second week of half days if she had a rough time.

I had been taking two thawed and one frozen bag (3 oz. each) of breastmilk to daycare for her; I recently increased that to three thawed and one frozen bag of breastmilk because Lila is a *snacker* instead of taking a lot at one time. That will probably change when we introduce solid food in the coming weeks.

If you can afford it, I highly recommend easing the baby into daycare part time a few weeks before you go back to school or work. It's useful to work out kinks beforehand – it is comforting to know that I'm right around the corner during those practice runs. A part of me felt really guilty doing this because I was home without the baby I got so used to caring for - so it's important to make good use of that alone time. I also feel 'mom guilt' often and that's not easy sometimes.

I have thought about the possibility of quitting breastfeeding because I've heard the stress of work can deplete your supply but I don't want to be overly stressed about when to stop. We will continue to do it until it no longer works for one of us.

It was hard to leave her those first few days and often still is. I cried far more than she did when I left her on that first day – I literally cried all day long – it was terrible! By day three, I didn't cry as much. This week I almost started crying again when I dropped her off because I'd had her home with me over the holidays and it felt like I was starting daycare for the first time all over again. Sleep deprivation (and we've had a lot lately) tends to bring on the waterworks easier too. Thankfully Lila smiles now when I drop and pick her up. She enjoys playing with the other babies.

AUTHOR'S NOTE

I met Christeen at a Breastfeeding Support Group. She had experienced and overcome a lot of issues with a very colicky baby. She is an intelligent warrior of a woman and the group and I are grateful for the many things we have learned from her. It is not just Christeen's students who do their homework.

REFERENCES:

Chapter 2
Ramsay DT, Kent JC, Hartmann RA, Hartmann PE. Anatomy of the lactating human breast redefined with ultrasound imaging. *J Anat*. 2005; 206(6):525–534.

Chapter 3
Abdoulahi M, Hemati Z, Mousavi Asl FS, Delaram M, Namnabati M. Association of Using Oxytocin during Labor and Breastfeeding Behaviors of Infants within Two Hours after Birth. Iranian Journal of Neonatology. 2017 Sep: 8(3).)

Lind JN, Perrine CG, Li R. Relationship between use of labor pain medications and delayed onset of lactation. J Hum Lact. 2014;30(2):167–173.

Condo DiCioccio H, Ady C, Bena J, Albert, N (2019.) Initiative to Improve Exclusive Breastfeeding by Delaying the Newborn Bath. Journal of Obstetric, Gynecologic & Neonatal Nursing. DOI: 10.1016/j.jogn.2018.12.008.

Chapter 4
Morton, Jane & Wong, Ronald & Y Hall, J & W Pang, W & Lai, Ching Tat & Lui, James & Hartmann, Peter & D Rhine, W. (2012). Combining hand techniques with electric pumping increases the caloric content of milk in mothers of preterm infants. Journal of perinatology: official journal of the California Perinatal Association. 32. 791-6. 10.1038/jp.2011.195.

Chapter 8
Harries, V & Brown A. (2019). The association between use of infant parenting books that promote strict routines, and maternal depression, self-efficacy, and parenting confidence, Early Child Development and Care, 189:8, 1339-1350.

Chapter 9
Goran MI, Martin AA, Alderete TL, Fujiwara H, Fields DA. Fructose in Breast Milk Is Positively Associated with Infant Body Composition at 6 Months of Age (2017). Nutrients 9(2):146.

Chapter 12
Morton J, Hall JY, Wong RJ, Thairu L, Benitz WE, Rhine WD (2009). Combining hand techniques with electric pumping increases milk production in mothers of preterm infants. J Perinatology (11):757-64. doi: 10.1038/jp.2009.87. Epub 2009 Jul 2.

INDEX:

About The Author

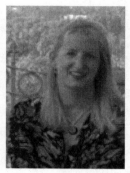 Mindy Cockeram graduated from Villanova University with a Bachelor's Degree in Communications in 1986. After relocating to London, England in 1990 and working for 14 years in the financial markets, she received a diploma from the University of Bedfordshire in Antenatal Education (2006) in conjunction with the National Childbirth Trust's (NCT' s) Teacher Training College. She taught for both the Wimbledon & Wandsworth Branch of the NCT and St Georges Hospital, Tooting SW20.

On the way to an NCT antenatal class in Wandsworth in 2009, she stumbled upon a woman in labor in a parking lot and delivered the baby. "I knew there was a reason for that coincidence and that I was in the right line of work" she said in an interview with London's ITV News.

In that same year as the 'car park birth', Mindy and her family relocated to Southern California where she certified with Lamaze International. She teaches childbirth education both privately and for a large hospital organization several times a week in the Inland Empire. She posts evidence based research articles on her Facebook site (learn4birth.com) and has a website of the same name: www.learn4birth.com.

PUBLISHED ARTICLES INCLUDE:

The Purple Line for Assessing Cervical Dilation.
https://www.lamaze.org/Connecting-the-Dots/Post/the-redpurple-line-an-alternate-method-for-assessing-cervical-dilation-using-visual-cues. Oct, 2012.

7 Classic Pregnancy Myths Revealed – https://www.lamaze.org/Giving-Birth-with-Confidence/GBWC-Post/true-or-false-seven-classic-pregnancy-birth-myths-revealed. Nov, 2014.

Co-author 'Raising Awareness Without Creating Fear – Teaching About The Perineum in Labour and Perineal Trauma', NCT Perspectives Journal, Issue 22, pg. 10-11, March 2014.

'Should I Stay or Should I Go Now' - When To Go To The Hospital Or Birth Center – BABE Series. https://www.lamaze.org/Connecting-the-Dots/series-brilliant-activities-for-birth-educators-should-i-stay-or-should-i-go-now-or-when-to-go-to-the-hospital-or-birth-center, June 30, 2015.

'What Can You Find in a Lamaze Class? A Ketchup Bottle?
http://www.lamaze.org/Giving-Birth-with-Confidence/GBWC-Post/what-can-you-find-in-a-lamaze-class-a-ketchup-bottle, June 14, 2015.

Fetal Surveillance – Alive and Kicking. https://www.lamaze.org/Giving-Birth-with-Confidence/GBWC-Post/alive-and-kicking-recognizing-the-signs-of-reduced-fetal-movement. July 5, 2016.

Not All Squats Are Created Equal. https://www.lamaze.org/Giving-Birth-with-Confidence/GBWC-Post/not-all-squats-are-created-equal-in-labor-birth. July 21, 2017.

Food For Thought in Early Labor & Beyond.
https://www.lamaze.org/Connecting-the-Dots/Post/food-for-thought-in-early-labor-and-beyond. May, 2018.

When Let down Brings You Down – Exploring Dysphoric Milk Ejection Reflex. https://www.lamaze.org/Connecting-the-Dots/Post/when-let-down-brings-you-down-exploring-dysphoric-milk-ejection-reflex-d-mer. August, 2018

UFO Doesn't Mean Unidentified Flying Objects Anymore: Labor Positions Activity – BABE Series. https://www.lamaze.org/Connecting-the-Dots/Post/brilliant-activities-for-birth-educators-ufo-doesnt-mean-unidentified-flying-object-anymore-labor-positions-activity, Sept 2018.

BY THE SAME AUTHOR:

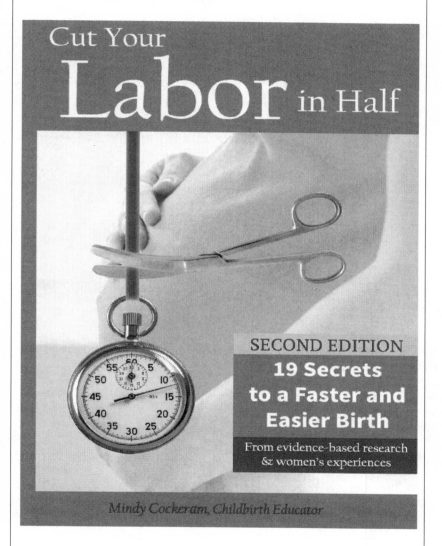

Cut Your
Labor in Half

SECOND EDITION

19 Secrets
to a Faster and
Easier Birth

From evidence-based research
& women's experiences

Mindy Cockeram, Childbirth Educator

Available at www.amazon.com

Made in the USA
San Bernardino, CA
12 April 2020

67632597R00117